MEREDITH O'BRIEN

Uncomfortably Numb 2

AN ANTHOLOGY
for Newly-Diagnosed MS Patients

W
Wyatt-MacKenzie Publishing
DEADWOOD, OREGON

Uncomfortably Numb 2
An Anthology for Newly-Diagnosed MS Patients
Meredith O'Brien

ISBN: 978-1-954332-58-4

Library of Congress Control Number on file

Wyatt-MacKenzie Publishing
DEADWOOD, OREGON

www.WyattMacKenzie.com

Requests for permission or further information should be addressed to:
Wyatt-MacKenzie Publishing
15115 Highway 36, Deadwood, Oregon 97430

Advance Reviews

"This follow-up to O'Brien's memoir, *Uncomfortably Numb* (2020), follows several multiple sclerosis patients and experts on their emotional journeys. It's easy to see shared experiences across the many narratives; many of the people presented here have faced similar challenges with aspects of their illness, from dealing with insurance and prescription drug cost issues to other people's judgement of using the American with Disabilities Act parking when their symptoms aren't visible to others. A project that many will find relatable."
— KIRKUS REVIEWS

"*Uncomfortably Numb 2* is a must-read for everyone living with multiple sclerosis—from the newly diagnosed to those who have lived with the disease for years, as well as people eager to learn more about MS. Meredith insightfully shares her experiences while also sharing the powerful stories of eight others on their respective MS journeys. This captivating book will educate, motivate and inspire all who read it."
— Dan and Jennifer Digmann, ACoupleTakesOnMS

"Meredith writes raw, candid stories of human vulnerability in the face of chronic illness. The experiences of different contributors including an artist, a social worker, and a pediatric neurologist show some of the breadth and variability of MS. It's a must-read for anyone facing the complex challenge of battling an illness and dealing with family dynamics, health insurance bureaucracy, workplace/disability accommodations, and everything else most take for granted. She strikes a balance between personal resilience and leaning on others, covering topics ranging from when to disclose a diagnosis to battling 'what if' questions about the future. No doubt people diagnosed with MS in the modern era can expect to live productive, fulfilling lives. The book also dabbles in politics, and we learn how health care policy affects us in ways we might not have considered."
— Brandon Beaber M.D., neurologist and author of *Resilience in the Face of Multiple Sclerosis*

"Meredith beautifully balances information with vulnerability! This book would have been an amazing resource for me when I was diagnosed in 2008. While my diagnosis story and experience is quite different I still found this book so helpful in processing my own MS journey."
— Jodi Dwyer, MS Activist, MSW, LICSW

Dedication

This guide is dedicated to the visionary Sylvia Lawry who, in seeking to help her brother with his multiple sclerosis, launched a movement by establishing the foundation upon which the National Multiple Sclerosis Society would thrive.

LIST OF CONTRIBUTORS

Elissa Grossell Dickey
COMMUNICATIONS & MARKETING DIRECTOR,
NOVELIST: RELAPSING REMITTING MS

Dianne B.
FORMER LIBRARY AIDE,
MS SUPPORT GROUP CO-LEADER: RELAPSING REMITTING MS

Sarah Quezada
FORMER CUSTOMER SERVICE AND WAREHOUSE SUPERVISOR,
MS SOCIAL MEDIA INFLUENCER AND ADVOCATE: RELAPSING REMITTING MS

Paige Butas
FORMER IT SYSTEMS ANALYST, FORMER ENDURANCE ATHLETE,
MS SOCIAL MEDIA INFLUENCER: RELAPSING REMITTING MS

Eddy Tabit
SOFTWARE PROFESSIONAL, NATIONAL MS SOCIETY BOARD OF TRUSTEE MEMBER
AND MS ADVOCATE: RELAPSING REMITTING MS

Lydia Emily
MURALIST, ARTIST, AUTHOR: PROGRESSIVE MS

Noelle Connolly
FORMER LICENSED CLINICAL SOCIAL WORKER,
RECREATIONAL BOXER: SECONDARY PROGRESSIVE MS

Laura Hoch
ASSISTANT VICE PRESIDENT FOR STATE ADVOCACY AND POLICY
FOR THE NATIONAL MULTIPLE SCLEROSIS SOCIETY

Dr. Tanuja Chitnis
NEUROLOGIST SPECIALIZING IN MS AND PEDIATRIC NEUROLOGY

Table of Contents

Foreword

Imagine you wake up one day and you can't see out of one eye. After a battery of tests, blood draws, and maybe even a spinal tap, you find your sitting across from a neurologist and you hear them say, "You have multiple sclerosis."

"Multiple what?" you utter. Hopefully the doctor gives some additional details and offers some soothing words before exiting and leaving you to figure out the next steps. And then, you likely take to your favorite search engine, or ChatGPT, to see what the internet has to say about your diagnosis.

This hypothetical vignette captures the experience that thousands of individuals experience every year when they learn that they have multiple sclerosis, or MS, which is a complex and unpredictable disease of the central nervous system, affecting nearly three million people worldwide. It can cause a range of symptoms, including fatigue, numbness, balance issues, and vision problems. While there are treatments available, there is currently no cure for MS. But don't let that discourage you from reading on. This book you hold (or are listening to) offers a wealth of insights and support for anyone affected by MS and those who love or want to support a person living with the disease.

I'm Dr. Tim Coetzee and I have the privilege of serving as the president and CEO of the National Multiple Sclerosis Society in the United States. Our organization was founded in 1946 by Sylvia Lawry after she and a band of individuals gathered in New York City and determined to do something about MS. At first, they focused on fundraising to support research, then they started raising awareness, advocating for more involvement in MS research by the federal government. Today our organization is devoted to finding a cure for MS and empowering those affected by the disease to live their best lives.

In my work, I have had the privilege of meeting many remarkable individuals who are part of the global MS movement. Meredith O'Brien is one of those individuals. I first met Meredith through her engagement with the Greater New England Chapter of the National MS Society. Meredith's journey with MS and her dedication to advocacy have been a source of inspiration for me and others in the MS movement.

I'm often asked to give advice to those who are newly diagnosed about what they should expect in a life touched by MS. I typically provide my perspectives, based on thirty-plus years in the MS movement as an MS researcher and a senior leader at the National MS Society, and point them to resources I think can be helpful. *Uncomfortably Numb 2* is one of the resources I'll now suggest. It is a comprehensive guide addressing different aspects of living with MS. From getting diagnosed to seeking emotional support, from requesting accommodations, to advocating for MS causes, this book covers it all. The beauty of this book is that Meredith has gathered contributions from various individuals—people with the disease, a neurologist, an advocate and more—who share their personal experiences of MS, providing a diverse and relatable perspective on the disease.

Meredith's reflection on her own diagnosis and the lack of relatable resources available at the time emphasizes the importance of sharing experiences to provide comfort and guidance to newly diagnosed patients. This sets the tone for the book, highlighting the unpredictability and challenges of living with MS, and the need for a supportive community. Each section is filled with perspectives ranging from grappling with the diverse ways MS can manifest as well as the different diagnostic journeys one can experience and the emotional impact of receiving a diagnosis. You'll explore the complexities of disclosing an MS diagnosis to family, friends, and employers, balanced with the importance of emotional support from family, friends, support groups, and online communities and so much more.

If you've made it this far in the foreword, I urge you to continue reading this book and join in traveling the MS journey with Meredith and the other contributors. This book is essential reading for anyone who wants to fully understand the journey of MS from the perspective of those living with the disease. Whether you are newly diagnosed, a loved one, or simply curious, you will find valuable insights and support in these pages. You are not alone. Together, we are stronger than MS.

Tim Coetzee, PhD
Albany, New York

You Are Not Alone

This is the book I could have used when I was diagnosed with relapsing remitting multiple sclerosis more than a decade ago. While there were websites and some dry medically-oriented books about MS, there was nothing that spoke to me, that authentically gave me a sense of what MS, in all of its iterations, was like for the people living with it. There was nothing that said, *Hey, here's what a bunch of other people experienced and here's what choices they'd make if they had to do it all over again.* I felt lost on a scary island where, when I started to type, "Is MS" into Google, the search engine suggested the word "fatal" for me.

As I worked through the initial months, I was unsure about how to handle this unpredictable disease of the central nervous system which strips nerves of their protective lining (myelin) and interrupts its signals, like a busted phone charger that only works sometimes. Questions haunted me: *Will I get worse? Will my ability to work be compromised? Will I need a wheelchair? Should I tell people, and if so, what should I tell them? How will this affect my ability to parent my kids? Will my marriage be compromised by my condition? Will my insurance cover my medication? Wait ... HOW expensive is that medicine?*

Aside from the guidance on the National Multiple Sclerosis Society's website (*Disclosure: I serve on the Greater New England Chapter of the MS Society and actively advocate for MS issues with state and federal officials*), I found that my initial neurologist was ill-prepared and/or politely disinterested in fielding my questions about new symptoms that plagued me—like a loss of taste, my inability to tolerate heat, and how to cope with hot flashes, which worsened my heat intolerance. For a period of time, as a direct result of having my reports of symptoms dismissed, I questioned myself and my perception of my symptoms. Then I switched neurologists and felt as though I had finally found a partner who co-managed my disease with me, who took the time to listen, who worked collaboratively, and who didn't gaslight me.

It took me six years before I finally mustered the courage to attend an MS support group. Once I started attending, I regretted not starting sooner. It took me just as long to inform my employer that I had MS and to later ask for accommodations so I could continue to teach without falling ill with MS symptoms resulting from overheated classrooms. Fearful my career as a part-time faculty member teaching journalism would be negatively affected by my admission that I have MS, once the news was out, there was no discernable change for me at work. It took me a few more years to finally get involved in MS Society events, where I fundraised for the Bike MS team and volunteered at other MS events.

My three children, who were young teens when I was diagnosed, are now adults and have all graduated from college. Two are in the work world while one is in physician assistant school. When we discuss how my MS affected my ability to parent them, sure, there's some sadness about the way my disease restricted me in terms of my level of energy, my difficulty with stairs and inclines, and my inability to tolerate heat and humidity. I missed events, concerts, Red Sox games, and many a family barbecue in the summertime. But during my decade-plus of living with MS, they've matured into empathetic people who think about more than themselves. They consider others' abilities and don't take one's health for granted. In order to be inclusive, they've learned how to thoughtfully organize gatherings so we can all be together as a family.

The same goes for my experience with friends and family. My young nephews are extremely considerate of my needs and limitations, like making sure vehicles are cool before I get inside. They never exclude me or treat me like an "other," or like a sick person. My friends understand my physical and temperature needs and we just work around them. They don't make me explain why, during particularly busy periods, I have to cancel attending an event or gathering. They've lent me their firm grips and their strong shoulders to help me limp through heat and humidity in order to get inside air conditioned venues so we can spend time together, and they never complain. They are boundlessly gracious and helpful.

Perhaps, I thought, *other folks could benefit from my experience.* Or, more accurately, my publisher thought this and floated the idea of this anthology to me. I then ran with it.

New MS patients can learn not just from my experience, but from the experiences of MS patients who live with very different versions of the disease. As I'm sure you know, the symptoms with which patients grapple depend upon which areas in the brain and spinal cord the MS has damaged, so multiple sclerosis looks different for each person. To capture a larger range of stories, I reached out to patients who you'd never guess had a chronic illness if you saw them at a party, as well as folks who use mobility devices to not just get around in their daily lives, but to travel widely. Some MS patients are athletes and others are vocal, passionate advocates for MS causes. Throughout these pages, I'll share their stories, and their thoughts on what they wished they'd known when they were first diagnosed. Those who offered up their stories include MS patients from across the United States: an artist, a recreational boxer, social media influencers, a novelist, an MS support group co-leader, a former triathlete, and a software company professional. I also collected stories from a top Boston area neurologist who specializes in MS and pediatric MS, as well as from a lobbyist who advocates for causes important to multiple sclerosis patients.

Here is some basic information that will help you understand the stories contained in this anthology.

Clinically Isolated Syndrome

The criteria necessary to diagnose MS has shifted over the years as disease experts have learned more.

When I was first suffering MS symptoms in 2012, conventional thinking was that if a patient experienced MS symptoms but an MRI only discovered one lesion (areas of nerve damage in the brain or spinal cord) and the patient had only had one "attack," that person didn't have MS yet. Instead, the person was urged to come in periodically for MRIs to see if anything changed and asked to report if they experienced new or worsening symptoms. Today, someone who experiences MS symptoms and has lesions on the brain or spinal cord—indicating damage to an area of the central nervous system preventing signals to flow properly—that person may receive treatment that could "delay or prevent a second neurologic episode and, therefore, the onset of MS," according to the National MS Society.

Symptoms which could indicate that there is MS-related damage to the protective nerve lining in the brain and spinal cord include: problems with vision, muscle spasticity, dizziness, walking difficulties, weakness, numbness, fatigue, and bladder and/or bowel issues.

Dr. Tanuja Chitnis, a neurologist who specializes in MS and pediatric MS at Brigham and Women's Hospital in Boston, said physicians are "a little bit faster diagnosing MS" now because of the fine-tuning the MS medical community has done to its criteria for establishing an MS diagnosis, referred to as the McDonald Criteria. The latest update, proposed in 2024 at an international convention of MS specialists, offered neurologists new testing tools to utilize alongside MRIs to diagnose the disease, the first stage of which is called Clinically Isolated Syndrome, characterized by an attack of symptoms in multiple timeframes and at least one lesion.

Relapsing Remitting MS

Most of the interviewees in this book live with a form of MS called relapsing remitting MS. The National MS Society says eighty-five percent of the one million American MS patients have this diagnosis, where patients experience "new or increased symptoms" followed by remission periods where "all symptoms may disappear or some symptoms may continue and become permanent."

Secondary Progressive MS

Now that there are ample disease modifying therapies (DMTs) available to treat the disease, fewer of those who are initially diagnosed with relapsing remitting MS go on to develop secondary progressive MS, where their symptoms continue unabated and worsen, with no remission periods. Prior to the availability of MS-specific DMTs, it was estimated that about half of relapsing remitting MS patients would develop secondary progressive MS within a decade of diagnosis. There is currently no reliable timeline or percentage of patients who may transition to secondary progressive.

Primary Progressive MS

Between ten and fifteen percent of MS patients receive a diagnosis of primary progressive MS. This means that a patient's symptoms, from the very beginning, do not go into remission. Instead, as the National MS Society says, "If you have [primary progressive MS], you will experience gradually worsening neurologic symptoms and an accumulation of disability."

Uncomfortably Numb 2

An Overview

Uncomfortably Numb 2—a sequel to my 2020 memoir about the first three years of my MS experience—will not offer any magical advice or perfect solutions to a disease that didn't have any widely-used treatments until the 1990s. Neither I nor any of the folks whom I quote know exactly what you're experiencing. We don't have miraculous answers for what to do in the event that certain symptoms crop up. Instead, the goal is for readers to benefit from the collective wisdom found in these pages. Newly-diagnosed patients, who most certainly are grappling with fear of the unknown, hopefully will feel like they have a community that is willing to help them and willing to listen, a community that will not insult them with misinformation like: *If you just eat purple foods on odd-numbered days and stand on one foot while you brush your teeth, you'll get rid of your MS vertigo and maybe even cure the disease altogether.*

Each chapter begins with my personal story, followed by other MS patients' stories, as well as input from a neurologist and a professional lobbyist for the National Multiple Sclerosis Society.

Just so you know that I'm not bluffing about this "I'm here to help you (but not in a medical way with any medical advice)" business, here's my website: mereditheobrien.com (don't forget the "e" in the middle). It lists ways to reach me. Drop me a line. If you have questions, I'll reach out to my network of MS-connected people to try to track down answers if indeed there are answers. In the meantime, just know that you are not alone. I repeat, for those in the back: **You are not alone.**

CHAPTER ONE

Getting Diagnosed

Getting Diagnosed

◆

Meredith

WRITER, LECTURER, MS ADVOCATE: RELAPSING REMITTING MS

I thought I was losing it. The stress of getting ready for a new job, of raising three middle schoolers had to be the culprit for the numbness that was creeping up my left side. Oh, and the anxiety—with which I'd struggled but had under control—must've contributed to my growing unease about the numbness that spread from the left side of my abdomen down to my left ankle. That's what a neurologist at a respected Boston hospital told me when I saw him in the fall of 2012 after two MRIs revealed I had damage, a lesion, on my brainstem.

Several weeks before this Boston visit, my primary care physician and I discussed the diminished sensitivity I'd been experiencing all summer, curling around my body like a weed. After ordering blood tests to discern if I perhaps had Lyme disease since there are a lot of ticks in New England, she also ordered an MRI.

"MS?" I asked her.

"Yes," she replied. "We'll wait and see what the blood tests and MRI say."

I was driving home from orientation for my new job teaching writing and journalism at a Boston area university, excited about my new career prospects, when her office called with the results. Not wanting to be driving when the news was relayed, I pulled off into the first parking lot I saw, clenched my stomach, and braced myself for the results. The nurse on the phone told me the MRI found a "mass" on my brainstem, not cancer, she said, likely MS. Nothing makes you feel as though you're gonna hurl like the words "mass" and "brain" used in close proximity to one another. The nurse said my physician wanted me to book an appointment with a neurologist but they had no recommendations for whom I should see.

Freaked out, I slowly drove home. It was the word "mass" that ignited a rapid unspooling of all manner of nightmarish scenarios in my mind, of all the horrible possibilities. When I got home, I started searching MS online, starting with the National Multiple Sclerosis Society because, of all the possible sources I could consult, certainly they would be able to give me the straight scoop. At that time, the site described MS by saying it is "an unpredictable, often disabling disease of the central nervous system that disrupts the flow of information within the brain, and between the brain and the body." It continued: "The cause of MS is still unknown—scientists believe the disease is triggered by as-yet-unidentified environmental factors in a person who is genetically predisposed to respond. The progress, severity, and specific symptoms of MS in any one person cannot be predicted." The site explained how the disease is categorized as an autoimmune ailment because one's own body attacks the protective lining of the nerves in the brain and spinal cord, interrupting normal communication between nerves, resulting in any number of ailments, which form a rogue's gallery of horribles: fatigue, walking difficulties, numbness, spasticity, vision problems, bladder problems, pain, cognitive changes, and on, and on the list went.

If I wasn't numb before I read through that site, I was when I closed my laptop.

Later, I had to open that laptop again in order to find a neurologist. I knew no one who routinely saw a neurologist and I had no idea what to look for, or what I'd need. So I picked a large Boston hospital with which I was familiar, looked up physician names on its Neurology Department page, called the office, and asked for the next available appointment with a neurologist. Once the consultation was scheduled, a second MRI was booked, this time with something called a contrast dye, which is injected into one's veins halfway through the MRI. This only amplified my tension as I'm claustrophobic. During the first brain MRI, I had moments of panic when my head was immobilized on each side by headphones which were slid into place by a lab tech, and then barricaded behind a hard plastic thing that is actually called a face cage. Because that's what a claustrophobic person needs, to be loaded into a narrow tunnel while her head is pinned in by headphones and a face cage inches from the tip of my nose. With my eyes squeezed tightly closed, I tried to maintain my composure during that first scan, to not have a panic attack, and to not have to squeeze the emergency get-me-the-hell-out-of-here bulb the tech placed in my hand and told me I could use to signal that I needed to get out of this frightening machine that enveloped me with noisy magnets that offered a nightmarish soundtrack.

The second MRI, weeks later, included a new feature. Halfway through the roughly half-hour scan, I was ejected from the machine like a disc from a CD player and had an IV clumsily inserted into the crook of my right arm so the contrast dye could be administered. Because I flinched when the tech inserted the IV, which resulted in my leg flinching as well, the tech harshly scolded me for moving. In that moment, all the emotion and fear I'd been compartmentalizing since the words "multiple sclerosis" were uttered, flooded out of me in the form of ugly crying. I felt humiliated that strangers saw my naked, emotional vulnerability. I couldn't even wipe the tears from my face because I was confined by a face cage and moving was forbidden. Knowing that the techs could see me via strategically placed mirrors was a shattering feeling of emotional exposure as tears slipped down my face and saturated my hairline.

Weeks later, my husband Scott—my college sweetheart from our University of Massachusetts at Amherst days—and I were in the neurologist's office for an evening appointment, after a full day of classes for me and work for Scott. I was tired and hungry and edgy as I dutifully and thoroughly gave the neurologist my medical history which included an experience with Bell's Palsy in my twenties (half of my face was numb and sagging for nearly two weeks, but it went away on its own), and my history of anxiety, the birth of my three kids following infertility treatments including one round of IVF. I was a newspaper and investigative reporter for years, so I prided myself on being thorough and exacting.

The neurologist, whom I guessed was in his late thirties or early forties, spent most of his time speaking with and making eye contact with Scott as he conducted the physical exam, as he checked my reflexes, as he watched me walk, and had me touch my index fingers from my nose to his finger in front of me. The most frustrating part was when he used a small pin to poke me on my extremities as he asked me to tell him, on a 100-point scale, how much sensation I experienced. As a word person, I had difficulty assigning a numeric value to the level of sensation I had at various spots. The journalist in me was uncomfortable with making up numbers on such an expansive, 100-point scale on the fly. What I knew for a fact: certain areas had less sensation than others and I could identify where those areas were. But that wasn't what the neurologist wanted from me. He wanted me to play by his rules.

The moment when he rendered his opinion was memorialized in my memoir, *Uncomfortably Numb*:

> His determination: I have one lesion on my brain stem. He says he has no idea how old the lesion is, but the MRI did not show it to be active. In fact, the MRI didn't show any additional lesions. "Multiple sclerosis is multiple lesions," Dr. Sabine (a pseudonym) says. He continues: "MS doesn't usually present like this. You have an unusual pattern of numbness that doesn't really conform with multiple sclerosis." He looks to Scott and nods affirmatively as if this all makes sense. In a pleasant, friendly voice, Dr. Sabine tells me to keep up with the yoga I am doing, urges me to de-stress myself, and to see him in January. As I walk out of there, I know I should feel relieved, but I don't. I get the distinct feeling that he doesn't believe that I'm experiencing numbness. Shame fills me as my face flushes.
>
> Years later, I read Dr. Sabine's medical notes from our initial meeting and they confirmed what I felt in the room. Despite the fact that the MRI found a "single lesion in the c-spine," described as a "hyperintense lesion in the central/anterior spinal cord at the C2 level, just below the cervicomedullary junction, approximately 10 mm in length," and that a physical exam found "decreased sensation to pin," Dr. Sabine wrote, "she does have a history of anxiety with panic attacks, and has been under significant stress recently; a psychosomatic manifestation is a strong possibility. The lesion noted on the brain/cervical spine imaging is unlikely to be related to her numbness."

At the follow-up in January 2013, I told Dr. Sabine that I had new numbness on my left hand; he brushed aside my complaints and told me to come back in a year "if anything new crops up," as though I hadn't just informed him of a new development on my hand.

In the ensuing years, the criteria for diagnosing MS has evolved to include something called "Clinically Isolated Syndrome." Using the frequently updated McDonald criteria—named after a New Zealand neurologist—patients need to have either multiple attacks and at least one lesion, or multiple lesions and at least one attack in order to be diagnosed, according to the UK's MS Society. Those who meet the McDonald criteria for having "Clinically Isolated Syndrome" are now prescribed disease modifying medication to slow the disease's progress, to reduce the number of attacks or "flares," and to slow down or halt the development of new lesions. "[S]tarting to use an MS drug as early as possible may be better than letting MS run its course," the American Academy of Neurology said in an April 2018 press release unveiling a revision of the MS diagnostic guidelines. "This is because the disease is known to get worse over time. According to the [new] guideline, several MS drugs have either strong or moderate evidence to support their use for slowing certain disease processes."

It wasn't until I experienced multiple attacks over the course of two weeks in July 2014—one which resulted in me being hospitalized for two days after being carted out of my house by EMTs—when I was finally diagnosed with relapsing remitting MS by an MS neurologist at the same Boston hospital. I had reached out to him a month before the attacks, when the left-sided numbness returned. This time, the reduced sensation went from my ankle to my chest and was accompanied by a tingling and radiating heat waves. And while I'd experienced the most stressful period of my life to that point—my 65-year-old mother died from a fast-moving cancer, my 67-year-old father was falling to pieces, and my full-time contract at the university where I was teaching wasn't renewed—I felt certain this was distinctly *not* a byproduct of anxiety. The MS neurologist administered the same exam Dr. Sabine had given me.

"She does have slightly decreased range of rapid alternating movements of the left arm," Dr. Walker (a pseudonym) wrote in my medical notes. "Light touch, vibration, temperature, and pinprick are all normal except for decreased pin in the whole left leg, the torso mainly in the back, less in the front. She has decreased temperature sensation in the left upper and lower extremities."

He sent me on my way with an order for a new MRI and an appointment to return in four months. He hesitantly handed me a glossy folder for newly-diagnosed MS patients.

Weeks later, my family of five had flown from Boston to Los Angeles for a much-needed ten-day vacation in a rented bungalow in Santa Monica which didn't have air conditioning. On our first full morning, Dr. Walker called saying he had my MRI results and wanted me to immediately come to the hospital. I was livid because I had called his office repeatedly before we left for the trip, begging for the MRI results but I was told they weren't available. (This was before the age of patient portals where patients can see the test results, sometimes before the physicians who ordered them.) I scheduled an appointment to see him on the Tuesday after my family returned to Boston. Dr. Walker never explicitly told me I had MS. Instead, he told me I had several new lesions, including one that was "enhanced," meaning that, at the time of the MRI two weeks prior, it was actively inflamed. When I hung up the phone, I think I must've been in shock, because I didn't ask if I should do anything differently between then and the appointment. Had I done so, had he given me some guidance, every horrific thing that happened after that could have potentially been avoided.

What is the "everything" that happened? Having Hollywood Bowl employees use a wheelchair to take me from the upper level of the arena where my family's seats were for a performance of pieces from Pixar films, to the first aid station on the first floor while my terrified children trailed behind. I had started violently vomiting, my limbs were weak, and I had trouble standing. I was intensely dizzy and had a painful burning sensation in the back of my head. In hindsight, it would've been helpful for me to know that some MS patients—including me, I'd soon learn—react this way when they're in heat and humidity. Had I known this, I wouldn't have spent ten days in an overly-warm Santa Monica bungalow without air conditioning. I wouldn't have hung out at the beach, or on hot city streets, or in steamy venues like the Hollywood Bowl on a July evening. On our final day in Los Angeles, I couldn't get out of bed, couldn't stand, was incredibly weak and dizzy, and couldn't stop vomiting and dry-heaving. My family packed up all our things, as we had to leave the rental by 11 a.m., and we went to Palisades Park where we had a view of the Pacific Ocean. We didn't know that the worst place for me to be was lying in the grass in the heat and humidity. We didn't know I was experiencing one, long, severe MS attack that rendered me, in the words of my then-15-year-old daughter, "looking drugged."

Some thirty-six hours after we arrived home, even in our air-conditioned house, I became terribly ill with vomiting, intense back-of-the-head pain, dizziness, weakness, and an inability to walk. I was carried down the stairs on a stretcher and taken, via ambulance to a local hospital, as my children again watched in horror. I was transferred to the Boston hospital where my neurologist worked (although he wasn't on call and no one from the hospital reached out to him). By the time I was discharged after two days on the neurology floor, I was sitting in Dr. Walker's private, suburban office and officially informed that I had MS. He said I needed to consider DMTs as soon as possible and handed me a stack of brochures from a variety of pharmaceutical companies explaining their MS medications. A few weeks later, after a new MRI, I learned that I'd developed more lesions on my brain and spinal cord and that one in my cerebellum was inflamed. Dr. Walker prescribed me three days worth of hospital-administered steroid infusions to stop the inflammation.

Knowing what I know now, if I had the opportunity to reboot this diagnostic process and do it again, I would've found a neurologist who specializes in multiple sclerosis from the beginning. The National Multiple Sclerosis Society's website enables patients to input their zip codes to find neurologists who "have demonstrated knowledge and expertise" with MS and "address the needs of those living with MS by coordinating multi-disciplinary care."

If I was able to go back in time, I would've reviewed patient assessments of potential neurologists because I now know that a physician's willingness to engage with and not patronize patients, is vital.

Given the technological advances and the digitization of medical records, it's now possible for patients to access MRI and other test results in their online patient portals, something that could've been helpful to me prior to my family's ill-fated California trip. If in 2014, I had access to my MRI results showing I had multiple new lesions, I would have demanded to speak with Dr. Walker and sent him emails via the portal. All the suffering and trauma inflicted on my kids as my husband anguished about what to do and whether he should've put our children on the plane back to Boston while he sought medical care for me could've been avoided.

Had I still gone on the trip, knowing the MRI results, I wish I had asked Dr. Walker if I had MS and if so, what I needed to avoid doing, or should do, during my family's Los Angeles trip. There's no need for feeling as though you're bothering your neurologist when something like your health is at stake.

In hindsight, it would've been a good idea for me to go to a Los Angeles hospital either on the night of the Hollywood Bowl attack or on the day my family was slated to fly home. A steroid infusion at that moment might have spared us the multiple ambulance rides and the fear it instilled in my three young teens.

Getting Diagnosed

◆

Elissa

COMMUNICATIONS & MARKETING DIRECTOR, NOVELIST: RELAPSING REMITTING MS

In 2004, a 25-year-old South Dakota newly-engaged journalist experienced sudden intense headaches accompanied by the blurring of her vision. After seeing her doctor, Elissa Grossell Dickey said an MRI scan revealed she had a single lesion in her brain. Two neurologists suggested that lesion could indicate that she had MS but, since she only had one of them, they couldn't definitively confirm the diagnosis. Get follow-up MRIs, they advised, and live your life. Though she was scared, Elissa said she planned her wedding and moved ahead with her marriage, had children, built a career, and traveled while she and her husband always kept in mind the sentiments of the song he sang to her when she was first diagnosed, "Come What May" from *Moulin Rouge*.

Nine years later, she woke up with no feeling in her left foot.

"At first I thought it was a running injury, but it spread up my leg, and then soon spread to my other foot and leg," Elissa said. "Sometimes I even struggled to walk due to muscle spasticity. But I still stubbornly felt that it couldn't be MS. They'd told me I didn't have it, after all."

This time, however, the MRIs were definitive and the diagnosis was clear. "It was such an emotional, scary time," she said, noting that the official diagnosis was conveyed to her in what she characterized as a "casual" manner by one of the medical professionals she encountered, although most, she added, handled it with care.

In spite of her fear, Elissa, now the mother of young children, said she felt a sense of relief to finally have an answer for what was causing her array of symptoms. "It had been several frustrating months of uncertainty and tests to rule things out, so it was a relief to finally receive a diagnosis," said Elissa. "I was feeling better by that time and had regained full mobility, so they even determined that I didn't have to start treatment if I didn't want to." She was given the option of monitoring the disease progression via MRIs to determine when or if she'd start taking disease modifying therapies (DMTs).

Looking back at the years-long process of figuring out what was wrong with her, Elissa said she now wishes she'd been a stronger advocate for herself, that she'd asked "more pointed questions," and demanded to be seen by physicians earlier. "If anything, I would give myself more grace."

To newly-diagnosed MS patients, or to those who think they may have MS, something that can be difficult to properly diagnose, Elissa said: "Don't be afraid to get a second opinion, to ask questions, to follow up after the appointment as needed. It also helps to have someone along who can listen to the information and ask questions as well."

Getting Diagnosed

◆

Dianne

FORMER LIBRARY AIDE,
MS SUPPORT GROUP CO-LEADER: RELAPSING REMITTING MS

Unlike Elissa's nine-year odyssey from initial onset of symptoms to her MS diagnosis, former Massachusetts public library employee Dianne B. said it took three days from the appearance of her symptoms for doctors to determine she had multiple sclerosis.

Dianne, then in her late thirties, woke up on the July 4 weekend in 2013 with profound numbness on the right side of her face which she said felt "like when Novocaine wears off." That numbness also encompassed her right nostril and part of her chin and featured a "pins and needles" sensation.

"I thought I slept on it funny and that it would go away on its own," Dianne said. "I remember attending a few barbecues with friends and family and I was worried that I was drooling because I couldn't feel the side of my face. My family assured me that I looked totally fine so I brushed it off."

The next day, an intense migraine piggybacked atop the strange facial sensations. Her primary care physician was concerned enough to send her to the emergency department, fearing Dianne was having a stroke. Many hours and several tests later, a physician told her that while the MRI ruled out a stroke, there were "some abnormalities," which were suspected to be Lyme disease; Dianne was given a neurological appointment for the following day, on July 6. Dianne remembers the neurologist telling her she had MS as he gestured to her MRI, which she said showed "my brain lit up like a Christmas tree. I never noticed any symptoms before the diagnosis," she said. "To me, it came out of the blue."

The suddenness of it all was jarring. "I was stunned and a little defensive at first, campaigning for the Lyme disease diagnosis, like I could bargain my way to a different diagnosis," Dianne said. "After all, I didn't know anyone with, or anything at all about, MS."

Her story isn't unique. Many people are unfamiliar with the disease or hold misconceptions about it even though it's estimated that nearly three million people worldwide have it.

Getting Diagnosed

◆

Sarah

FORMER CUSTOMER SERVICE AND WAREHOUSE SUPERVISOR,
MS SOCIAL MEDIA INFLUENCER AND ADVOCATE: RELAPSING REMITTING MS

For Sarah Quezada, her diagnosis happened "exactly 100 days before my thirtieth birthday, on July 22, 2012." The mother of two very young children whom she had "back-to-back," Sarah said her initial symptoms were varied and easily attributed the general fatigue of working full time as a customer service and warehouse supervisor in California who had a baby and a toddler at home.

"The morning I went to the emergency room I had stood up from bed to grab my son and I just completely face-planted on the floor," Sarah said. "I couldn't feel my left leg at all."

In hindsight, she said she realized there were signs that something was off but she never acknowledged those signs. "I was making a ton of mistakes at work, swearing I had returned that email, completely blanking on calling someone back," Sarah said. "When I would walk out back to the warehouse, it would take me forever" to reach her office. And she was told her gait was noticeably lopsided.

She was not okay.

After a full day in the ER led to her being admitted, she said she endured a battery of tests which eventually landed her in front of the on-call neurologist who matter-of-factly told her that she had MS, an incurable, sometimes debilitating disease; he then casually asked if she had questions.

"My husband is great at asking questions," Sarah said. "He always thinks of things to ask that I never do. He had left about an hour earlier to go get our kids from my sister. In that moment, the only thing I could think to ask was if I was going to die from it."

Informed that she wouldn't die from it, a pair of nurses who were in her room at that moment sat down on the bed on either side of her. "One held my hand while I cried and the other rubbed my back," she said. "Neither acted like they had anywhere else to be. I'm not sure how long they actually stayed with me, but it was the kindest thing for them to do."

Getting Diagnosed
◆
Paige

FORMER IT SYSTEMS ANALYST, FORMER ENDURANCE ATHLETE,
MS SOCIAL MEDIA INFLUENCER: RELAPSING REMITTING MS

Utah endurance athlete and IT systems analyst Paige Butas was in her late thirties when she was overcome by a "bad headache." She said that headache "turned into a numb spot on my head that spread down the entire right side of my face over the course of a week." She was experiencing dizziness, memory problems, and what she described as "auditory hallucinations," things she'd never had.

The neurologist she consulted suggested she could be experiencing MS symptoms. However, he added that the criteria for diagnosing her with multiple sclerosis, was "very conservative."

Paige said: "He told me, 'If it is MS, it's not a matter of if but when you have another episode. There is still a chance all of this was caused by stress.'"

According to the National Multiple Sclerosis Society, seventy-four percent of MS patients are female and most are diagnosed between the ages of 20 and 50. Women with autoimmune diseases—who vastly outnumber male patients—often have their symptoms dismissed by physicians as a result of anxiety. Over forty percent of women "eventually diagnosed with a serious autoimmune disease" had been considered "a hypochondriac," said the founder of the American Autoimmune Related Diseases Foundation.

It would take four years for Paige's "maybe you have MS" to transition into a definite diagnosis. She said she began struggling with a constellation of symptoms that her colleagues noticed and then told her they were afraid she was having a stroke. She wasn't. It was MS, something her neurologist confirmed for her over the phone saying, "Where you have now had a second episode, I am confident in diagnosing you with MS."

Getting Diagnosed

◆

Eddy

SOFTWARE PROFESSIONAL, NATIONAL MS SOCIETY BOARD OF TRUSTEE MEMBER
AND MS ADVOCATE: RELAPSING REMITTING MS

It was April 1, 2009, the day after his thirty-sixth birthday, when New Hampshire software professional Eddy Tabit noticed something awry with his vision. "It felt like I stared at the sun and then tried to read my computer screen," he said. Some three months later, Eddy, a very active and athletic person, had numerous tests including MRIs, and was told he had relapsing remitting MS.

The neurologist who gave him this unwelcome news then "used scare tactics to make sure I started medication, predicted I would not be able to work in three to five years, and I would possibly not be able to walk in the future," Eddy said. "[The] doctor explained that I had a black hole," which refers to an area of the brain where the damage to the nerve protective covering, the myelin sheath, is permanently destroyed.

"I remember breaking down in tears in the parking lot with my wife," he said. "We were expecting our third child at the time—my wife was six months pregnant—so it added to my fears."

Getting Diagnosed

◆

Lydia
MURALIST, ARTIST, AUTHOR: PROGRESSIVE MS

California muralist and artist Lydia Emily didn't have insurance in the mid-2010s when she was worried she was having a stroke. A battery of symptoms which sent her to the ER numerous times had been plaguing her over a period of months: mysterious shoulder pain, burning toes, a neck that felt as though her "head was on a spike," she explained in her 2024 book *The Art of Hope*. When her symptoms didn't dissipate, she was urged to seek psychiatric treatment.

On a December day in 2012, Lydia said she could no longer speak, move her tongue or open her eyes because the pain in her head was too intense. At this point, an MRI was finally ordered. This test, whose results were delivered to her by what she described as an uncomfortable-looking ER physician, put to rest any hypothesis that Lydia Emily's problems were psychosomatic. They were symptoms of an aggressive form of MS.

"At that moment," she said, "I felt bad for my mother who was clearly very upset, and for the ER doctor who felt so bad about giving me the news."

Getting Diagnosed

◆

Noelle

FORMER LICENSED CLINICAL SOCIAL WORKER,
RECREATIONAL BOXER: SECONDARY PROGRESSIVE MS

New Jersey-born Noelle Connolly's health problems began when she was in boarding school in Massachusetts, and experienced trouble with her feet and legs. The 17-year-old was rehearsing for a school play, *The Music Man*, when she noticed tingling sensations in her feet which eventually started spreading up her legs past her knees. She even got accidentally pushed off the stage during rehearsal. While walking the streets of Boston with her visiting parents who were in town for her play, she said she felt strange, but ultimately didn't do anything about it after a school nurse suggested the feeling was likely due to a potassium deficiency.

Days later, Noelle's discomfort turned into pain. "I noticed that the pain had become so uncomfortable that I could no longer walk on my feet," Noelle said. "It felt like I was walking on glass, that I had knives being stuck in the bottom of my feet. It was excruciatingly painful."

After an unproductive ER visit in the Boston area, Noelle was sent home to New Jersey where she was seen by her pediatrician who referred her to a pediatric neurologist. While she was in the neurologist's waiting area, she said, "I saw this man watching me as I was walking to the bathroom because I could hardly walk on my feet. I was in so much pain. We went in [to the exam room] and he said he saw me walking and was watching my gait." He didn't offer her an MRI but he did something Noelle described as "nerve testing" to which the results were inconclusive. Noelle and her mom were informed she either had MS or was "a dramatic, 17-year-old blond girl." Weeks later, when her foot pain subsided, Noelle returned to school and faced a fire-hose of rumors from classmates that she'd been faking her symptoms. And since she had no diagnosis to offer as an explanation for her absence, she didn't know how to respond to the gossip.

Noelle's symptoms worsened. Knowing what she knows now, Noelle said things she thought everyone experienced—like intense fatigue, feet which experienced fiery jolts and later the stabbing sensation of icicle-sharp cold, her tendency to get really sick, numbness, and "an electrical storm in both my legs ... like lightning shooting off" after exercising—were actually indications that she had MS.

By 2005, the symptoms seemed to be increasing; she lost the ability to control her left hand, so she again sought medical help. Finally, a suburban neurologist suggested a cervical spine MRI, followed a few days later by a brain MRI. The 23-year-old was taking her Chihuahua, Mr. Martini, on one of their daily, five-mile walks when the neurologist called and told her she likely had MS. She was no longer being dismissed as an overly-dramatic young woman. "I guess I was happy because I finally was going to get a name of what was going on with me, but at the same time, how was this going to change my life?" Noelle asked.

However, when the neurologist was reluctant to put Noelle on any medication to potentially stop the disease progression, her mother stepped in and got her a referral to an MS clinic in Boston. Being seen in a specialized clinic made the difference, Noelle said. Her diagnosis was confirmed, her feelings were validated, her description of her symptoms was taken seriously, and they crafted a treatment plan. She said the team showed her "that I still could live a pretty productive and great life."

Getting Diagnosed
◆
Dr. Tanuja Chitnis
NEUROLOGIST SPECIALIZING IN MS AND PEDIATRIC NEUROLOGY

Once named a *Boston Magazine* top doctor, Dr. Tanuja Chitnis manages roughly five hundred MS patients at Mass General Brigham in Boston, one hundred and fifty of which range in age from 10-17. Her practice is part of a group of a dozen pediatric MS centers around the United States. She knows the challenges of not just diagnosing MS but of diagnosing it in young people because its symptoms can mimic those of other ailments. "There's always a period of, 'Well, MS doesn't happen in children,' even though we've worked really hard to combat that misguided notion," Dr. Chitnis said.

Fitting a young patient's symptoms together like pieces of a puzzle isn't always straightforward. If a child has started falling often, for example, parents and pediatricians may think the child's falls are the cause of a weak leg, not that the child's leg is weak and that is causing the falling, she said.

"It is a really tough diagnosis in a young person, I think, for anyone, but especially when you're a teenager and it usually hits in high school," Dr. Chitnis said. "These young people are struggling with high school as it is, and then now, a new diagnosis. And there's always that period of adjustment. Even if we can diagnose it quickly, getting them onto a treatment can take some time."

She estimated it takes her patients six to twelve months to adjust.

An important aspect of the diagnosis is that she can encourage her patients to be hopeful. She informs the patients and their parents that "they can continue with their school, their college, have a job. They can have a family if they wish to."

Dr. Chitnis said it's important to her that her patients are encouraged to be hopeful. Her message is: "I want you to know that now we have very good treatments for managing MS. We're going to put you on the right treatment for you. Young people who have a diagnosis in this era do very well."

CHAPTER TWO

Telling People

Since you may have very different reasons for disclosing to different people in your life, your explanation needs to be tailored to the situation and the particular person. And because no two people are alike, no two responses to your disclosure are likely to be the same.

– The National Multiple Sclerosis Society website

Telling People

◆

Meredith

WRITER, LECTURER, MS ADVOCATE: RELAPSING REMITTING MS

For someone who has always been fond of being the first to tell people the latest news—a trait I apparently demonstrated even as a young girl, so I guess I was destined to work in journalism—I uncharacteristically did *not* run out and tell everyone after I was diagnosed with multiple sclerosis. In 2014, the National MS Society's website urged MS patients to use caution when divulging one's diagnosis to people, given that many people don't fully understand what the disease actually is. (I was one of them prior to my own diagnosis.)

My 67-year-old father, who was in the throes of mourning my mother's death, initially had difficulty understanding MS when I told him I'd been diagnosed. He was clearly of the view that MS was always fatal. When we'd talk on the phone, he'd insert an air of urgency into his voice, "How *ARE* you?" as though I was perpetually *thisclose* to the grave. When he didn't hear from me when he thought he should have, he assumed it was because I was in the hospital again with another MS attack. It took years for him to finally understand the complexity, the unpredictability, and the fluctuations inherent in this disease. A decade into my MS diagnosis, he now understands a bunch of my symptoms, especially my fatigue and heat sensitivity, and isn't as panicked as he was for years. Knowing someone with MS will do that.

But worrying about people jumping to the conclusion that I was on death's door because they didn't understand MS wasn't the only reason that I held back on disclosure. At age 45, I was concerned about how people would see me, worried they'd do that sympathetic, squinty thing people do with their eyes or make micro-adjustments to their tone of voice as if they're speaking with a child. I didn't want to be perceived as sick or less capable. I was prideful in that way. I wanted to still wear clunky and chunky heels and to not look like there was anything at all wrong with me.

However.

I now realize, that was unrealistic. And shortsighted. I underestimated a lot of people.

Outside of a small circle of friends and family, I didn't widely share the news. I didn't share it on social media and I didn't write about it. This, I later discovered, left people to speculate why I wasn't at a lot of my three kids' games (they were three-season athletes) especially on hot and humid days, why I didn't attend a few parties during particularly busy times of the year, why I was largely unable to work all day and then go out at night, and why I didn't wake up early to drive my kids to school or make them breakfast. During one Open House event at their high school where parents are supposed to follow their child's schedule and there's precious little time in between classes for us to get to the next class, it happened to be an unseasonably warm evening. I started to feel ill due to the heat and had struggled with so much walking up stairs—as I didn't know where the elevators were and was too embarrassed to ask—that one father made a wisecrack about how slowly I was going.

During one Christmas season I had a surge of energy and stupidly threw myself into doing far too much so that by the time I was attending a holiday concert in which my elder son was performing, I slumped against a wall, unable to stay on my feet, worried my legs were going to collapse. I looked like a person who'd had too much to drink and decided to ask Scott to take me home. Even though I really wanted to see that concert, I worried people would think I was drunk or drugged or disinterested. I fretted constantly that people would think I was a slacker of a mother—I *am* a GenXer, the "infamous slacker" generation—that I was lazy, that I was uninvolved, that I was unsociable ... any negative inference folks could draw when noticing my lack of participation or attendance to kids' events caused me to worry about their perceptions.

So I started to share and to educate. I tried to nonchalantly drop into conversations and on the sidelines of games little tidbits of information about MS. To those attending awards events in hot gyms where I found myself pressing ice packs and cold beverages to my neck and face, I explained heat sensitivity. I devised a quick go-to explanation: MS is like having a frayed phone charger that only kind of charges if you wiggle it around a bunch. But sometimes it just doesn't work at all. MS does that to nerves in your brain and spinal cord, messes with the messages they try to send. Depending upon the symptoms with which I was struggling, I would explain that the nerves involving my temperature regulation or my ability to climb stairs were affected. (The fatigue thing is harder to explain as many people live under the delusion that they get it because they're tired, too. Not. The. Same.)

When I heard my young nephews characterize my MS as "something wrong" with my brain—they weren't wrong, I just hated the way it sounded. So I explained, in a basic way, how MS worked. Today, two of them are teens and one is in his 20s, and they have a good understanding of the disease and how it affects me.

My biggest concern was for my career and whether or not to inform employers about my MS. My university lecturer contracts were issued on a semester-by-semester basis, so I feared if I told the people in my department at the large university where I taught that I had an unpredictable, incurable disease of the central nervous system that they'd drop me, figuring why would they want to waste time with someone who could have a flare-up or have her condition go south on a moment's notice?

A year after my diagnosis, when I applied for the lecturer post I currently have, the application material included a form entitled "Disability Status: Voluntary Identification of Disability." There was a long list of ailments, including multiple sclerosis. Applicants were directed to check off one of three boxes: that they do not have a disability, that they previously *had* a disability, that they currently have one of the listed disabilities, or they choose not to answer. I checked, "I do not wish to answer," which was, essentially, saying that I have one of the listed disabilities. Would they, if they found out, stop asking me to teach classes? Would they think that I'm less capable than others? That I was a risky hire, particularly if I inquired about any longer-term positions?

Eventually I had to tell them. Why? Well, in 2020 my memoir, *Uncomfortably Numb* was published. Up until that point, the people for whom I worked had no idea that I had MS. And even if I hadn't had that memoir published, I would still have had to tell them I had MS during the COVID pandemic because I requested to teach remotely for one semester longer than the university wanted. Because I am immunocompromised and take immune-modulating medication for MS, I formally filed a request (which was granted) to teach via Zoom during the fall of 2020—before vaccines were available—because I worried I'd be vulnerable to becoming very sick. (Which was a good move because, when I contracted COVID in December 2022, after keeping up-to-date on all my vaccines, I became severely ill, reaching a temperature of 104.7. Imagine what would've happened had I gotten sick in 2020, prior to having received any vaccinations.)

Overall, while the majority of people's eyes widened with fear when I initially told them about my MS, they seemed to take their cues from me, from the tone I used as I explained it. If I didn't act panicked or overly solemn, they didn't either. I was, and remain, fairly matter-of-fact about it all. This is how I live my life now, how I move through and engage with the world. I'd rather have people know what's going on than jump to conclusions.

The National Multiple Sclerosis Society's website has an abundance of advice on everything from whether you should tell your employers ("disclosure in the workplace can have a significant impact on your job security, employment options, and career path"), your friends ("no need to tell everyone at once"), and even folks you're dating ("While there's no need to tell all on a first date, remember that secrets don't lay a very good foundation for a lasting relationship"). You need to determine what works best for you.

Knowing what I know now, if I were diagnosed today, I don't think I'd worry so much about telling people I had MS. I'd be more open. The more people know and understand about the disease, the better.

I wished I'd embraced the role of educator as I shared with friends and acquaintances what was going on. Maybe that would've made life easier for my younger son when I couldn't help him as much as I wanted to after his siblings left for college. (They'd previously been able to drive him around and help me out.)

As for whether informing my employers that I have MS has affected my job status? All I can say is that they continued to offer me classes and asked me to be the department's writing coach. During a couple of semesters, I was asked to teach the equivalent of a full-time load. They didn't ask me, however, to teach full-time. Whether that was a matter of funds, of my skill set, of their needs, or of my chronic illness, I'll never know.

Telling People
◆
Elissa
COMMUNICATIONS & MARKETING DIRECTOR, NOVELIST: RELAPSING REMITTING MS

Elissa kept immediate family and her closest friends updated on what was happening after she received her diagnosis, but it was hard. "It wasn't always easy to talk about," she said. "Sometimes I thought I could tell someone about my diagnosis without any problem, but the moment I spoke, I started crying."

The reactions this South Dakota resident received tended to, overall, be "wonderfully kind," but she said there was an undercurrent of questions and uncertainty rooted in people's lack of understanding about what multiple sclerosis is. Some folks offered her untruths from the internet, like the person who suggested the reason she developed MS was that Elissa drank diet soda. "The first time it happened, it really caught me off guard and it was unsettling," she said. "Now, though, I'm able to brush it off."

Elissa, whose novel *The Speed of Light* features a character who's given an MS diagnosis, said she's open about her MS journey with people, but sometimes doesn't have the bandwidth to handle the range of reactions she receives. "In general, I've never hidden my diagnosis," she said, "... But there have been times when I didn't feel like I had the mental space or emotional capacity to tell someone. Sometimes it's because I feared they would have a bad reaction, either downplaying it or offering a well-intentioned but unhelpful 'solution,' like the diet pop situation. Other times, it was because I feared my own emotional reaction when saying it."

She also said it can be challenging when well-meaning people try to compare one person's experience with MS to another and expect them to be the same. One person wanted to introduce her to someone else they knew who had MS because that individual was "so positive about it." Elissa wondered if this implied she wasn't handling her diagnosis well. "I really do try to stay positive as much as possible, but I definitely don't need any toxic positivity in my life."

For those who've recently received their own MS diagnosis, Elissa said, "Your story is yours and the way you tell it is your own. So if one day you're an open book, and the next day you don't want to talk about it at all, that's absolutely valid and okay."

Telling People

◆

Dianne

FORMER LIBRARY AIDE, MS SUPPORT GROUP CO-LEADER: RELAPSING REMITTING MS

Within the first week of Dianne's diagnosis—which occurred a mere three days after the onset of symptoms—she had contacted family and close friends by phone and email and took time off from work for medical appointments including a second opinion. Once her MS was confirmed by a second neurologist, Dianne shared the news online.

"The one benefit to being diagnosed, and to my great relief, is I found out how many people love me," she said. "Have you ever wondered who would attend your funeral? Those few weeks after my initial diagnosis were like a living funeral. Friends and family mourned the loss of my previous life, of the person I was before the MS attack, and they were all scared and uncertain of the person I would become."

While no one "abandoned" her afterward, nobody in her circle had any experience with the disease so it was a steep learning curve for everyone. "The first few months involved a lot of them Googling and sharing any article or information they could gather to send me," she said.

Always an independent person, Dianne, who lives in central Massachusetts, said the diagnosis upset her because it made her "feel weak" as well as annoyed her because she didn't want to inconvenience anyone. When friends and family offered help, she tried to refuse it, denying she needed it, but they helped her anyway. "If it weren't for their love, I'm not sure where I would be today," she said. "I am so lucky to have this support. I know my situation may not be the norm, so I appreciate my friends and family every day and am thankful they didn't allow me to push them away like I tried to so many times."

To those who've recently received an MS diagnosis, Dianne offered this advice: "People are going to share everything they know or heard about MS with you and sometimes what they share is not helpful or even true! I have one friend who sends me any article or story that mentions or hints at a cure for MS, even if the info was unhelpful. I always thank them for thinking of me and tell them I will take a look because I know they have good intentions and just want to help."

Telling People

◆

Sarah

FORMER CUSTOMER SERVICE AND WAREHOUSE SUPERVISOR,
MS SOCIAL MEDIA INFLUENCER AND ADVOCATE: RELAPSING REMITTING MS

Sarah has for years maintained a website and lively social media accounts under the name MSfitMomma, so it might not come as a surprise that she shared her MS diagnosis online while she was still in the emergency room.

"I process things by talking about them, so early on, I started a blog to help share my story and help me process it," Sarah said.

Sarah's employers already knew what was happening, she said, given that she was undergoing "intense physical therapy to learn how to walk again," which kept her out of work for a few weeks. However, her family couldn't afford her to be out of work, so after a month, she tried returning to the workplace. It didn't turn out so well. Her body rebelled. She wound up being out of work for another four months.

"My job was so understanding and helpful," Sarah said. "When I went back to work, we tried to have me do my job that I had held for ten years as customer service and warehouse supervisor, but it was just too many moving parts, so they gave me the job of receptionist. It felt degrading at the moment, but I knew they were just trying to help me out. It was before Obamacare, and I needed a job with healthcare."

Additionally, major MS attacks sent her to the hospital for two separate stays, resulting in the need for more physical and occupational therapy.

Although she was living her experience out loud, Sarah said for several years she "did a bad job accepting" her diagnosis. "I felt mad and sad and frustrated. I couldn't take my kids places by myself because a walker and two toddlers was too much to handle."

Most of the people in her life had lovely and polite reactions to news of her diagnosis. One of her mother's close friends—an "auntie"—sat with her when she was in the hospital so she wouldn't be alone. Sarah could only recall one reaction to the news that "stung" and it was from a person who was close to her who she said "started telling people that she thought that my husband was going to leave me now that I was disabled. I was stunned. She knew us both well."

In spite of that, Sarah has been open with her children about what is happening with her MS.

"I decided early on that because my MS was so physical, that I was going to explain it to my kids once they started asking questions," she said. "I told them that your brain gives your body directions and the 'holes in my brain' were like I hit a pothole. Both of my kids at different times have replied to a question about me using a walking aid because I have 'holes' in my brain."

Telling People

◆

Paige

FORMER IT SYSTEMS ANALYST, FORMER ENDURANCE ATHLETE,
MS SOCIAL MEDIA INFLUENCER: RELAPSING REMITTING MS

Paige initially limited the circle of those who knew about her diagnosis to her close family and, even with them it was "just the basics." The Utah IT systems analyst told her then-boss about the MS diagnosis simply because she needed to obtain steroid infusions for several days and had to leave work early.

"I did not tell my coworkers for another year," she said. "I was always afraid of the stigma that came with being chronically ill. Everyone I knew saw me as a strong, inspiring athlete, and I wanted to keep that persona alive."

News of Paige's MS proved stunning to many of the people she told: "I was super active, super healthy, at the peak of my fitness. So this was pure shock all around. My dad and brothers were very concerned and my husband was quietly panicking. No one in my family, or myself, really knew what MS was."

When she learned she had MS, she was a self-described "serious endurance athlete." But her triathlons had to be sidelined for the first year after the diagnosis, something which affected a few of her friendships. "The people I thought were my friends, I guess we were only friends because of our commonality," she said. "When I couldn't train or race anymore, all of those people disappeared."

Like Elissa and Dianne, she received her share of suggested "cures" from people and encountered numerous conversations with people who didn't understand the chronic, incurable disease, including asking if it would imminently kill her or when she'd "get better."

Her advice to the newly-diagnosed: "Share what you are comfortable sharing. Just be aware not everyone in your life will be understanding or accepting."

Telling People

◆

Eddy

SOFTWARE PROFESSIONAL, NATIONAL MS SOCIETY BOARD OF TRUSTEE MEMBER
AND MS ADVOCATE: RELAPSING REMITTING MS

Eddy didn't tell his family about the testing or suspicions that he might have MS until it was official. When he knew for sure and told them, many of his family members wept.

"I remember my sister crying," he said. "It was hard to think that her big brother was sick. My parents also cried but also wanted to know exactly where I was going for treatment and if I was getting the best care." Eddy and his brother joked because "that's how we interact."

With friends, he said sharing the news seemed "a bit tricky."

"It's awkward to call people just to tell them you've been diagnosed with a disease," he said. "I looked for ways to bring it up with friends I saw frequently."

The diagnosis, like with Paige, surprised people who saw Eddy as fit and healthy.

"Most friends were shocked because they looked at my physical appearance and it didn't make sense to them," Eddy added. "I have always been very active and exercise regularly. To them, I seemed in better shape than most people they know."

While people were polite, he said, there were some who asked if this diagnosis meant he was going to pass away soon. Some people suggested diets and treatments that would "fix" his MS symptoms.

Looking back, Eddy said he regrets not informing some of his friends, as there were a few who didn't find out about his diagnosis until years later.

"I should have found a way to reach out sooner," he said.

Telling People

◆

Lydia
MURALIST, ARTIST, AUTHOR: PROGRESSIVE MS

Lydia wasn't at all hesitant about sharing her diagnosis.

"I'm pretty sure I told everyone," she said. "My village was very supportive. Lots of hugs and concern and offers of help."

A single mom with two young daughters, she called her kids on the phone from the hospital to let them know what had happened.

For newly-diagnosed patients deciding who to inform about their disease, the California artist said: "The only advice I can give to anyone is to be patient. Those who love you will fumble and make mistakes, but will do everything they can. Those who don't you can let go."

Telling People

◆

Noelle

FORMER LICENSED CLINICAL SOCIAL WORKER,
RECREATIONAL BOXER: SECONDARY PROGRESSIVE MS

Because Noelle was diagnosed at such a young age, she had to date while having a chronic illness. She first met the man who would become her husband, Christopher, when they were in the same English class at a Massachusetts boarding school and briefly dated during their senior year.

"I broke his heart and he ended up going to Denver University and I ended up going to Lesley University and living totally different lives for about eight years," Noelle said, adding that she eventually reconnected with Christopher after she'd come out of a serious relationship. By the time they went to dinner for their first date as adults, Noelle was very sick and in the midst of chemotherapy as an off-label treatment for her MS because she said her MS symptoms were out of control. She told Christopher: 'You would be crazy to date me because I am a disaster and a mess.' And I truly felt that way. But he didn't. It didn't bother him."

When Noelle underwent the chemo, she had to do it in the hospital because she was allergic to it and had adverse reactions. Even though they were a very new couple, Christopher was there during one of her treatments when she had the allergic reaction. Noelle's mom fled the room because it was so upsetting for her to witness. Christopher, Noelle said, came into the room and "just looked at me and said how beautiful I was. And that was it."

But not everyone is Christopher.

"Telling people all depends on, I think, the situation, the person, the place, the time, and where you're at in the diagnosis," she said. "I think there is a time that sometimes I wish I was a little bit more quiet about it, but at the same time, I wouldn't be where I am now."

When Noelle told her fellow twentysomething friends she had MS, she explained that it was similar to living with the flu. "Some of my high school friends couldn't really grasp and understand what MS meant, especially because, at that point it was relapsing remitting, so it wasn't in their face," she said.

One encounter with a high school classmate a few years ago disturbed her. That classmate was working as wait staff at a restaurant and, when she saw Noelle enter with her family while using a walker, she hid from Noelle. Weeks later she called Noelle saying she had in fact seen her and knew about her diagnosis, and said "her heart was broken when she saw me with the walker and saw how much I required assistance in my walking. And she said in that moment, my diagnosis of MS became very real for her, even though she had known this, even though she had known that I was diagnosed in 2006 because I wasn't using a walker or wasn't having really true, active mobility issues at the time."

Noelle said society doesn't realize that some people's disabilities may be invisible, like hers was before her MS symptoms worsened. Now she needs mobility aids ranging from a walker and a cane, to a scooter and a wheelchair in order to move through the world.

"I can't hide my MS diagnosis any more because of my mobility issues," Noelle said. "So that means that my kids can't hide behind it, so they're amazing advocates and telling people that I have MS and I'm okay with that. And we've had many situations that they have had to advocate for me in public when people have made comments to us."

Telling People

♦

Dr. Tanuja Chitnis
NEUROLOGIST SPECIALIZING IN MS AND PEDIATRIC NEUROLOGY

For Dr. Chitnis's teenage MS patients, the question of who to tell is a frequent question as few teens want to appear different from their classmates. She encourages her teen MS patients to speak with the pediatric MS clinic staff including a nurse, a psychologist, a neuropsychologist to work through issues about revealing their diagnoses.

Her college-age MS patients, Dr. Chitnis said, "are maybe struggling with school. They're pretty open to [counseling help] especially realizing they want to make the most of their college years."

As for her adult patients and whether they should tell their employers about having MS, Dr. Chitnis said there are laws prohibiting disability discrimination. "There is less of a concern about telling your coworkers or your boss, however I think it depends on the scenario you have and specifically around the workplace," she said.

What advice does she give to new MS patients? "You can tell if you want to," Dr. Chitnis said. "You don't have to tell anyone."

CHAPTER THREE

Seeking Emotional Support

Seeking Emotional Support

◆

Meredith

WRITER, LECTURER, MS ADVOCATE: RELAPSING REMITTING MS

I like to joke about how my husband and I have been a couple since the Reagan administration. We started dating in 1988 when I was a first-year UMass-Amherst student and he was a sophomore. We got married in 1992 when we were mere babies—at ages 23 and 24 respectively. We've endured job changes and challenges, many moves (including one from Massachusetts to Maryland and back again), the death of beloved pets, the struggles and disappointments of infertility treatments, three miscarriages, raising three children (including a set of twins), the deaths of our mothers, and two serious heart afflictions, including a heart attack. By far, one of the hardest things with which we've grappled has been my MS diagnosis. It changed everything.

We had been a 50-50 kind of couple who divvied up household chores and collaborated on big decisions. We role modeled, as best we could, gender equality. When our kids were babies, Scott got up to change them in the middle of the night before bringing them to me so I could feed them. When they were still very young, Scott worked from home a couple of days a week—before COVID made working from home widely acceptable—so I could teach classes at a university. We had long-term aspirations for ourselves and for our family.

Then multiple sclerosis entered the chat.

Then fatigue settled over me like a dense fog, rendering me unable to tackle multiple big tasks or events in the same day without rendering me bedridden for the next twenty-four to forty-eight hours. A few months before I was diagnosed in 2014, we had attended a handful of theater performances, including one I'd been looking forward to seeing, starring Bryan Cranston in *All the Way* on Broadway; he won the Tony for that role. In spite of my anticipation for the performances, I kept falling asleep. I didn't know what was wrong, why I couldn't keep my eyes open. I was struggling with intense fatigue at work that several lattes couldn't overcome. Once I learned I had MS and finally received an explanation as to why I could pound down the caffeine but no longer push through events like I used to, our whole nightlife changed. I became someone who, in her forties, needed naps and had to pace herself.

Summers were irrevocably ruined. With my damaged brain and spinal cord unable to handle heat and humidity, I couldn't go to the beach unless it was cooler or later in the afternoon; otherwise, I would become ill, dizzy, and dry-heave. The only thing that stopped the reaction was to immerse myself in cold water. I couldn't attend outdoor events like Red Sox games, concerts, or family barbecues if it was too hot or humid. Long, hot summer days at Cape Cod left me, essentially, grounded inside air-conditioned locales so I wound up encouraging Scott to go out and do stuff. (I'd be lying if I didn't admit that it kills me that I can't join him. See more about this in Chapter Seven: Living With It.)

It's hard for any marriage to weather the ups and downs of life, but when chronic illness upends everything, that results in guilt (me), resentment (me worrying that he's resenting my illness, and me resenting the fact that he can enjoy things I can't any longer), and fear (the both of us, me about being a crappy wife who can't do what she used to, him about how we can move forward and live our best lives while my MS is still of the relapsing remitting variety).

While I can seek support from Scott—who can describe the minutiae of my daily MS experience and who's always looking to make things better for me, even if he can't "solve" my MS—I don't think it's fair for me to rely solely on him to be my emotional crutch. I can get frustrated with him for not *getting* it, for not giving me space for flare-ups of anger and pissed-offness because he wants to fix everything. It's what he does. He fixes things.

And I don't really put my full emotional weight of my MS experience on my friends, even the closest ones, even the ones who've helped drag me from an air-conditioned car in hot and humid weather to the air-conditioned museum, even the ones who have seen the after-effects of me having to endure heat and humidity. Don't get me wrong, I share with them my frustrations and my experiences, but not as in depth or in as much detail as I do when I complain about other things, like, why my kids are calling me a Boomer when I'm a GenXer, and why are the Red Sox owners making such bad trade decisions. Barring the earth-shattering discovery of an MS cure, my MS is going to shadow me for the rest of my life. It's not going away. There's going to be no end to my MS journey, so while I will share with my friends the latest developments, or perhaps mention that the humidity has really been getting to me lately, I'm going to seek the heavy-duty support elsewhere.

Where, you may ask? Well, I have an excellent therapist with whom I can share the purest version of my truth and since she doesn't have a vested interest in our relationship—she doesn't live with me or hang out at Red Sox games with me—I don't worry that I'm placing emotional burdens on her (more on this in Chapter Five: Getting the Help You Need). But other than the amazing therapist Kathleen, I have found that the most authentic places where I can seek support and share my own experiences include an online MS support group I joined during the pandemic, and social media and podcasts created by MS patients. I will admit that I was reluctant to join an MS support group because I initially didn't want to face folks whose MS had progressed further than mine, a seeming harbinger of my future. If there were people whose symptoms were more severe than mine, I figured, I wouldn't be able to be honest if I was "just" experiencing relapsing remitting MS.

When I was promoting my 2020 MS memoir in as many online venues as I could, because in-person book events were all canceled—thanks COVID!—I was invited to speak to the MS support group that was geographically closest to me. Prior to COVID, the group met in person, but after I spoke with them about my memoir, they invited me to join them and I figured I'd give their group a try. I found warmth, acceptance, wisdom, and a bone-deep understanding of the disease. It was okay to gripe with them, okay to say you were floundering, okay to be yourself. I didn't have to worry that I was unloading a dump truck-worth of emotional baggage on their heads. It was freeing.

As much as social media and the internet has coarsened our national discourse, spread misinformation, and deepened wedges in a politically polarized public, it has been an amazing source of comfort and support for those with chronic illnesses. Via blogs, Facebook, Twitter (RIP), Instagram, and Threads, I've "met" many people with MS. We've liked, shared, and commented on one another's posts. We've expressed our sadness when a treatment didn't work or when someone's MS worsened. We've cheered one another on when they tackled something new when we've had successes. I've appreciated how they share bitingly funny memes about MS and chronic illness that made me feel seen and heard. In fact, several of the folks whose posts have buoyed me, I've invited to contribute to this book.

If I could go back in time to the beginning of my MS journey, I'd absolutely look for and start attending an MS support group immediately. While my newly-diagnosed self would have seen people whose disease has progressed further than my own, which might have been a bit worrisome, the benefit of the camaraderie, the knowledge, and the humor of the folks in the group far outweighs the fears about what may happen with my MS. Those uncertainties will be there, regardless of whether or not I interact with people whose multiple sclerosis is more advanced than mine. Yes, when you first learn you have MS, the whole uncertainty business can be wildly daunting (for more on this see Chapter Seven). And it made sense that, out of a sense of self-preservation, I was trying not to expect the worst of the spectrum of MS symptoms to immediately manifest themselves within my body. I was trying to focus on the moment and not the future.

I urge new MS patients to follow social media accounts run by MS patients and organizations. I didn't do that initially because I was afraid to "out" myself online by being seen following these accounts, afraid that people who didn't understand what MS was would make negative judgments about me. That was silly. Just because someone follows someone on social media doesn't mean they, too, have a particular ailment. Maybe someone they know and love has it. Maybe they want to learn more about something. No one can make assumptions. The wisdom and sense of community at these sites is well worth it.

Seeking Emotional Support

◆

Elissa

COMMUNICATIONS & MARKETING DIRECTOR, NOVELIST; RELAPSING REMITTING MS

While noting that her husband, sisters, and parents provide the bedrock of her emotional support as she copes with a life with an incurable disease, Elissa said the most important coping mechanism she has developed has been creating plans to address her fears that may crop up.

"The best thing I learned was if I get trapped in the fear of the future, asking myself scary, 'what if' questions—such as, 'What if I find myself suddenly unable to walk again?'—I should answer those questions," she said, "come up with an answer, make a plan, and that will give it less power over me."

She also turns the negativity of those "what if" questions on their head. "What if everything works out perfectly for me?" Elissa said she asks herself. "That has stayed with me to this day and helps me when I get anxious about the future!"

Elissa advises newly-diagnosed patients to pace themselves in terms of how or if they seek support from others. "It's okay if you don't want to talk to anyone right away. It's okay to want to talk to someone one day and not the next," she said. "There's no right or wrong way to react, and no right or wrong way to seek support. If you prefer to talk to a friend, have an online chat with a counselor, visit a therapist in person, or attend a support group, all of those are valid choices. Do what works for you."

For Elissa, her first experience with a support group was a negative one where members pressured her to immediately start taking disease-modifying therapy even though she and her neurologist said she didn't need to rush. "I felt judged and didn't go back. Looking back now, I realize they were just trying to help, but it was intimidating for me when I was newly diagnosed," she said. Elissa said that now she feels confident in how she's navigating her multiple sclerosis and might one day consider returning to a support group.

Seeking Emotional Support

◆

Dianne
FORMER LIBRARY AIDE,
MS SUPPORT GROUP CO-LEADER: RELAPSING REMITTING MS

Dianne had the opposite experience when she sought guidance from an MS support group. In fact, she's now the co-leader of one in central Massachusetts. (*Disclosure: I attend Dianne's now-Zoom-based support group.*) Two months after learning she had MS, she showed up to an in-person meeting and wound up making "lifelong friends" with people who truly understand what it's like to live with this illness.

"I know my friends and family love and support me, but my MS friends understand what I'm going through and that makes me feel like I'm not alone in my MS world," she said. "They have walked, or rather tripped, in my shoes."

But Dianne says it's important for people to find a group with which they feel comfortable. "Finding the right support group is no different than finding your friends," she said. "Meeting new people can be intimidating but these are your people! They know what you're going through. They have felt what you feel. Not every group may be a fit for you, but keep looking."

As for how to seek support in coping with all the uncertainties of MS, Dianne suggested being very clear with friends and family. "I do my best to keep my outlook positive but sometimes I have bad days and need to just vent so that is what I do," she said. "If I am not looking for advice or solutions, I tell whoever will listen that I just need to unload. I say that I am having a pity party and it's going to be a rager!"

Clarity about your needs can help avoid miscommunication: "Be open and honest with your needs. Don't expect anyone to read your mind but at the same time, realize that not everyone will understand what you are going through."

Seeking Emotional Support

◆

Sarah

FORMER CUSTOMER SERVICE AND WAREHOUSE SUPERVISOR,
MS SOCIAL MEDIA INFLUENCER AND ADVOCATE: RELAPSING REMITTING MS

Sarah said the first support group meeting she attended met on a Tuesday morning and was held in a church. Most of its members were generations older than she was, a young thirtysomething, and the vibe didn't feel right for her. So, she left and created her own community online on social media.

Now, Sarah's Instagram account—MSfit Momma—has nearly 1,500 followers and that's where she said she found her voice and support.

She said her circle of loved ones lives by the adage: *When I got MS, we all got MS.* "I have a very large support group of family and friends. I know this is not the case for all people," Sarah said.

Sarah's friends and family have formed local Walk MS teams for National MS Society events over the years, something that made such an impression on her children. "My kids still call it the Orange Parade, even though they're teenagers now," she said. "The energy is like nothing else I've ever experienced."

Seeking Emotional Support

◆

Paige

FORMER IT SYSTEMS ANALYST, FORMER ENDURANCE ATHLETE,
MS SOCIAL MEDIA INFLUENCER: RELAPSING REMITTING MS

Paige's experience mirrored Sarah's in that she had a bad run-in with an MS support group so decided to create her own online community in 2022. "They were depressing for the most part, and I didn't feel I fit in," she said, "so I started posting content on TikTok in efforts to build my own community. At that time, TikTok was lacking in MS-specific content. I spotted the need so I ran with it."

Paige posts on TikTok under the name "msfighter101." Her informational videos sometimes focus on misconceptions about MS, but many of them feature her sharing info about the disease while she expertly applies makeup. As of the time of this writing, she had nearly 21,000 followers on the platform.

"The community grew very quickly and it has been the best thing for me with all the support and validation from others," she said. "... I remember how validating it was when I started communicating with others who were experiencing the exact same things I was, particularly from an emotional level."

Within her personal sphere, Paige said she seeks emotional support from her husband, but did so "unwillingly" at the beginning of her MS journey. "I am very stubborn and hard-headed, so asking for help is like pulling teeth for me," she said. Eventually, though, after working with a therapist in a neuro rehab clinic she said she began to understand how the neurological effects of her MS impacted her emotions. (She later created Tik-Toks about the topic of denial and MS.) "One thing [the therapist] taught me was living in the moment. The only thing you have control of is whatever is happening in that moment."

Nowadays, Paige said of her relationship with her husband, "Our connection has actually grown stronger since I started relying on him a little more."

Her advice for folks who are newly diagnosed? "Being strong doesn't mean taking on everything by yourself. Being strong means being willing to admit you need help, and accepting that help."

Seeking Emotional Support

◆

Eddy

SOFTWARE PROFESSIONAL, NATIONAL MS SOCIETY BOARD OF TRUSTEE MEMBER
AND MS ADVOCATE: RELAPSING REMITTING MS

For Eddy, his wife is his chief source of emotional support. "Occasionally, friends ... remind me that I should stay in the present and try not to worry about the future. Keep doing what works now."

His best advice to people who've just gotten word that they have MS: "Definitely talk with loved ones, but also find accurate information. Google searches will return doom and gloom. I looked for positive information (success stories with meds, people who are living normal lives, etc.)."

Eddy, who is active with the Greater New England Chapter of the MS Society (*Disclosure: I'm on the local Board of Trustees with Eddy.*), urges patients to utilize the well researched and vetted information offered by the National MS Society's website. "They present it in a way that provides hope," he said.

Seeking Emotional Support

◆

Lydia
MURALIST, ARTIST, AUTHOR: PROGRESSIVE MS

Lydia is all about leaning on family, including her two daughters, and friends.

"I know that my village has always been incredibly supportive," she said. "... Love, laughter, food. Support comes in all of these forms all the time."

Lydia, who has been a prominent advocate for the National MS Society, appearing in promotional videos and speaking at events, also gave a nod to the Society as a resource for support services.

"I don't wanna sound like I'm plugging anything, but the Multiple Sclerosis Society, or anything like that, is really helpful, information about drug information, about support groups," she said. "I found a lot of solace in that when I needed it."

Seeking Emotional Support

◆

Noelle
FORMER LICENSED CLINICAL SOCIAL WORKER,
RECREATIONAL BOXER: SECONDARY PROGRESSIVE MS

Even though she was trained as a professional social worker, Noelle said it "has taken me some time to figure out my support system and find people who I need and who I have allowed to be a part of my circle and my support system."

She counts her husband Christopher as her number one supporter: "He was very understanding and is one of my biggest advocates. He encourages me to spread my wings and to find the support system that I need to be able to thrive with this illness and in this life and anything that I need to do to be able to function as a mother, as a wife." She also said she appreciates her "amazing family support system" that includes her parents, brother, and her extended family, including her in-laws.

With years of therapy under her belt, Noelle said she felt comfortable co-running an MS support group through her physical therapist's office until COVID put an end to their meetings. "A lot of the support groups that I found in the beginning were people who had been diagnosed for a very long time, or were very angry," she said. "And because I was so young, they couldn't connect with me at all. And they kind of just scared me, and that's not how I was going to be."

What proved to be a vital source of emotional support for her? A Parkinson's boxing group. After her MS transitioned to secondary progressive, Noelle needed to boost her strength, found a boxing program for Parkinson's patients, Punch for Parkinson's, and asked if they'd let her participate. Her boxing coach has now become one of her biggest supporters. She told a Boston area MS infusion group, the Elliot Lewis Center, she "noticed an immediate improvement in my self-esteem and overall mental health. I was shocked and thrilled by the positive changes in my body. This experience taught me that it is okay to ask for help, to go out of my comfort zone, and taking a risk on something new."

In recent years, Noelle said, she's realized she needed someone to help her in her home.

"I need someone to help me around the house, and what I also figured out is, I don't need someone to just clean or help me make the beds or do my laundry," she said. "I almost need a friend and so I've been blessed to have a helper, Jackie, who is my right-hand woman. She is here to hold me up. She is here to make sure I put my medicine in my mouth. She is here to stick my canes all around me because she knows I walk around the house without my canes or without my walker."

Being picky about whom you include in your clinical care team, Noelle said, is something she highly recommends. "I want providers who want to be part of my team and are willing to allow me to be an active part of my care process," she said, adding that it's likewise important to remember that "it's okay to fire care providers" if they're not listening to you.

Seeking Emotional Support

◆

Dr. Tanuja Chitnis

NEUROLOGIST SPECIALIZING IN MS AND PEDIATRIC NEUROLOGY

Finding a community is vital for not just pediatric MS patients, but for their families, Dr. Chitnis said. In 2005, her hospital was one of the first centers in a group of six at the time for pediatric MS care. Mass General Brigham's pediatric MS program is now part of a network of over a dozen pediatric MS clinics that work together to increase awareness, conduct research, and to provide support.

"There is a community of parents and kids themselves, and also newsletters for pediatric MS, so there's a lot out there," Dr. Chitnis said. "There are camps as well for kids with MS to go to in the summertime. We've had events, especially prior to COVID, we had annual parent and family days, bowling events, and Red Sox games. Now it's transitioned to online programs."

CHAPTER FOUR

Seeking Accommodations:
At Work & Public Venues

Seeking Accommodations:
At Work & Public Venues
◆
Meredith
WRITER, LECTURER, MS ADVOCATE: RELAPSING REMITTING MS

Remember how, in Chapter Two, I mentioned that I was initially concerned about informing my supervisors at the university where I was teaching that I have MS? I was wildly concerned about being officially "out" as someone who lives with a chronic illness who also needs accommodations to be able to work. While employers are legally mandated to accommodate those with disabilities to give them what they need to do their jobs, I feared that because I was a contract employee—each contract was for the duration of a single semester—it would be so simple for the university to just not renew it because of the messiness involved with accommodating my needs, which mostly involved not teaching in an overheated classroom that would trigger my MS heat sensitivity.

Then COVID happened.

I felt required to apply for an accommodation in the fall of 2020 and the spring of 2021—before the advent of widely-available COVID vaccines—because I didn't want to be forced to teach in-person classes, which the university was encouraging at the time. "Upon just learning about the on-the-ground conditions under which faculty will be operating this fall semester, I have requested the ability to teach my two journalism courses remotely," I wrote in an email to human resources officials, something that felt akin to jumping out a small plane and hoping that the parachute opens. I included a letter from my neurologist written on hospital letterhead. "She is immunocompromised secondary to her disease and the disease-modifying treatment prescribed to combat her MS," my neurologist wrote. "She is advised to avoid any and all areas, including the work setting, which may expose her to the COVID 19 virus. She is not physically able to resist virus and infection, and it is dangerous for her to work in the suggested atmosphere for the 2020-2021 school year."

So there it was. The first, in-writing request for the accommodation I needed. Would this request put a bullseye on me, identify me as someone who is more trouble than she's worth? Apparently not, because I was kept on staff and remain on staff as I write this, albeit in a part-time capacity.

Not telling employers about one's multiple sclerosis and not asking for accommodations seems to be prominent among MS patients. An August 2022 study by the *International Journal of Environmental Research and Public Health* called "Stigma, Discrimination and Disclosure of the Diagnosis of Multiple Sclerosis in the Workplace: A Systematic Review" found that: "The prevalence of people with MS who experience some degree of stigma in the workplace can be as high as 79.2%. Those who report greater feelings of discrimination are more likely to be unemployed. The prevalence of employers' and co-workers' awareness of the diagnosis varies from 31.7 to 90.2%. The main reason for non-disclosure is the fear of being discriminated against. The psychosocial work environment needs to be taken into consideration as part of public and individual policies to promote the health of patients with MS."

I had to ask for another less official accommodation, the second semester when I taught in person as the university dropped mask requirements and regular COVID testing. The classroom to which I'd been assigned to teach a news writing class was cramped and the only person wearing a face mask was me. There was no way for me to maintain a six-feet distance from students. I couldn't maintain a three-foot distance. I reached out to my department administrator and she relocated the class to two separate rooms depending on the day. I felt incredibly grateful for the accommodation given that when I first contracted COVID in December 2022, after having kept up with my vaccines, I was incredibly ill. My temperature was nearly 105. I was hallucinating and my MS symptoms flared.

But it's not just in the workplace where I have experienced a growing compulsion to advocate for my own health. Keep in mind, I'm not someone who likes to be singled out, who doesn't want to ask for things, who doesn't want to make a fuss. I hate feeling as though I create a spectacle due to my physical needs. For example, I have an allergy to dairy products and it routinely mortifies me to have to be a pest to staff at restaurants as I ask them to alert whoever is preparing the food to make sure they understand the scope of my allergy. Hate. It. And when I'm served something with cheese on it, in spite of my warnings, I still feel badly when I have to alert the server to the error. To quote Taylor Swift, I'm a "pathological people pleaser."

However, in order to live my life, I need accommodations. Because I have experienced increasing difficulties trying to navigate the summer's heat and humidity—my legs weaken, my vision becomes impaired by flashing lights, and I am overcome by dizziness and nausea which prompts retching—I eventually applied for and received a disabled parking placard. Initially, I used it to limit the distance I'd have to traverse in order to walk from an air conditioned vehicle to an air conditioned venue like a store or restaurant, so the heat sensitivity symptoms wouldn't (hopefully) have time to emerge before I got to where I needed to go. When I use the placard, I'm always on the lookout for someone who would likely scowl at me for using it given that *knock on wood* my disease remains largely invisible to others, unless I'm curled over and retching.

It was during an "invisible" moment on a hot, humid fall day that I decided to park in a disabled spot at the university campus. The collective impact of commuting to the Boston campus, walking across campus (vigorously between the two classes so I wouldn't be late), teaching, returning to my car and commuting home, frequently resulted in me crashing into my sofa as soon as I got inside my house unable to do much else. I needed every shred of energy I could conserve in order to teach effectively so I didn't want to spend it by walking across campus, nevermind having my heat sensitivity triggered by unnecessary time in warm weather. On this particular afternoon, an older man stopped his sedan and shouted at me as I walked away from my vehicle, "Do you know that that's a handicapped spot you parked in?" This man, who used arm crutches to get around campus, shot me a look of disgust and shook his head when he saw me later that day.

Years earlier, another older man made me feel as though I was trying to cheat the system when I sought to use the handi-capped elevator at the Boston Garden instead of climbing the stairs to get to my seats at a U2 concert. After looking me up and down—I was wearing wedge sandals, apparently not what the elevator operator expected of someone who wanted access to an elevator—he said, "This is a handicapped elevator."

I told him I knew that, but that wasn't enough to stop his questioning stares. I felt compelled to fill the silence. "I have MS," I said as he, Scott, and I stood awkwardly in the elevator.

He paused for a beat, then asked, "Well do you have a card or something?"

"A card?" I asked. I'd never heard of an MS card. I later asked my neurologist who said there was no such thing.

Perhaps he meant a handicapped placard, I thought, *but that was left in the car.*

I shook my head, "No" and endured his silent judgment until we got to our seats for the Experience + Innocence Tour where I still had to climb a few stairs to get to our seats. One would've thought that the operator of the elevator for disabled people's use would've had the experience to understand that not all disabilities are immediately obvious. Instead, I felt as though I'd done something wrong.

Since those experiences, I've taken to sliding a print-out of the National MS Society's logo—with the words, "I have MS" hand-written beneath it—onto my dashboard to, hopefully, ward off any nasty-note-writing people because I don't fit their image of what a disabled person should look like. I've also become more accustomed to asserting, if someone questions me, that I need to use the elevator because my MS causes fatigue and impairs my ability to use stairs. But I'd be lying if I said going out in public and asking for accommodations I need is easy. Not for someone like me who doesn't like being singled out.

If you were to ask me what I'd do differently regarding seeking accommodations if I was able to speak to my newly-diagnosed self, I'd tell younger me to stop being so proud and to just get that disabled placard, to just ask for a classroom where it's not roasting inside, and to just use the elevators when they're available. Nobody cares if you do these things, save for random cranks who might ignorantly question you. (If my younger, newly-diagnosed self remained skeptical, I'd tell her to search online for the "I Have MS" business cards to flash to people—or just make her own—which'll make them back off.)

What difference did having these accommodations make to the quality of my life? Getting a handicapped placard enabled me to go out to dinner with my family at The Mad Minnow in Cape Cod in the middle of summer without having my appetite ruined by nausea and the wave of heat-related symptoms I endure. It allowed me to park close to the building where I was teaching during a recent semester so I wouldn't expend unnecessary energy moving myself to and from my car and would instead save the energy and focus for my students.

Using the disabled elevator at the Boston Garden allowed me to enjoy a Boston Celtics game with my nephews when we had nosebleed seats which still required me to ascend a few more stairs. It made it possible, when Madonna decided to start her Boston Garden show two hours late, to conserve my energy, make it to the end of the show, and be able to exit the building, and get to an Uber without my best pal Gayle having to drag an exhausted Meredith down the streets of Boston.

Ask for what you need. You'll be happy you did.

Seeking Accommodations:
At Work & Public Venues
◆
Elissa
COMMUNICATIONS & MARKETING DIRECTOR, NOVELIST: RELAPSING REMITTING MS

Elissa said she is lucky that her workplace is flexible and that she has not needed to "officially seek accommodations."

While she knows when she's out in the world she needs to be able to have a place to sit down and can't be in the sun too long due to her MS symptoms, Elissa said she hasn't felt the need to seek special accommodations at public venues.

"My husband is a strong advocate for me," Elissa said. "He'll make sure we have a shady spot and plenty of water in the summer, or in the winter, he'll drop me off at the door before parking at an event if it's icy because my balance isn't the best."

Seeking Accommodations:
At Work & Public Venues

◆

Dianne
FORMER LIBRARY AIDE,
MS SUPPORT GROUP CO-LEADER: RELAPSING REMITTING MS

"I worked at a public library when I was first diagnosed and had optic neuritis, which greatly affected my ability to read. I used a lot of text-to-speech applications to read and speech-to-text to write! I was allowed to use my mobile phone on the floor because it had applications like the magnifying glass to help me see."

In addition to using technology to help in the areas where the MS had caused her difficulties, Dianne decided to get a handicap parking placard the first summer following her diagnosis.

"Heat greatly affects me and can worsen my fatigue so I do what I can to conserve my energy," she said. "I use the pass to park closer to store entrances because otherwise walking across a hot parking lot would sap my energy and I wouldn't be able to complete any errands. Work smarter, not harder!"

When Dianne travels with her family to venues like amusement parks, for example, she said they "thoroughly research disability accommodations before we travel."

"If we can't find the information online, we will call before making the trip. If there is going to be a lot of walking, consider a mobility aid," she said. "If there is no shade, consider a sun umbrella. If it will be hot, consider cooling gear. Be prepared!"

She's a big advocate for not only asking for whatever help you may need so you can enjoy your trip, but for reading up about your rights, according to the Americans with Disabilities Act of 1990.

Seeking Accommodations:
At Work & Public Venues
◆
Sarah
FORMER CUSTOMER SERVICE AND WAREHOUSE SUPERVISOR, MS SOCIAL MEDIA INFLUENCER AND ADVOCATE: RELAPSING REMITTING MS

Sarah didn't have an easy time of it when she got back to the warehouse where she worked as a supervisor following her diagnosis. Because of the complexity of her supervisory role, her employers asked her to instead work as a receptionist, a move which she understood, but said still hurt her feelings.

She said this was in the days before the 2010 Affordable Care Act, which, after its passage, forbade health insurers from discriminating against people with preexisting conditions and enabled people to buy health insurance through state exchanges which cover essential services. When she was diagnosed, Sarah said she needed to keep her job in order to maintain her insurance coverage for her MS care.

When it came to accommodations, Sarah sought and received a handicapped placard at the behest of her primary care physician even though, at this point, her disabilities were not visible. "I got stares from older people because I was young" and using the handicapped placard, she said.

"One time, a man did shout at me to leave [the space] for someone else because I wasn't using a mobility aid that day," Sarah said. "I was walking into Target and was going to use the cart as a mobility aid."

Even when she has used her cane, she has had encounters with people who don't recognize her needs; like the woman who moved Sarah's cane without asking in a darkened movie theater. "I was caught so off guard that I didn't say anything to her in the moment, but I felt very violated," Sarah said. "For me, my walking aids feel like an extension of my body, so for her to reach down between my legs, essentially, was so uncomfortable."

When she's attending a concert or a sporting event at an arena or stadium, Sarah said she often calls in advance to speak with someone about the availability of ADA seats. "It is a hassle to get a hold of a human," she said. "The best advice I have is to be pleasant and charm them. We went to a [baseball] game for Father's Day and the lady couldn't get me ADA seats, but she spent a long time finding me the best seats in the section I could afford and good seats that I could walk easier to since I'd be using my cane."

Like Dianne, she also researches ADA rules and guidelines for any airline or park she and her family are planning to use.

"I have made it my personal policy to pull up the ADA accommodations rules for wherever we are going and that is how I learned that an amusement park we were going to for my son's birthday now requires a form you fill out at least forty-eight hours before you visit to be authorized by your doctor stating that you need ADA accommodations," Sarah said. "We could have gotten to the park and not been able to get the ADA line accommodation, which doesn't mean you cut the line, they give you a time to return which is the equivalent to the line wait time for everyone who waits in the line."

Even if they can be difficult to get, Sarah says accommodations are worth trying to obtain. "Accommodations are there to help make your day/trip/life easier. Don't be too proud to ask for them," she said. "Ask as soon as you know you are going somewhere that you will need them and call as soon as you buy your tickets to request them. Don't wait until it gets closer to request them."

Seeking Accommodations:
At Work & Public Venues
◆
Lydia
MURALIST, ARTIST, AUTHOR: PROGRESSIVE MS

Lydia used accommodations of her own making in the mid-2010s when her MS was starting to affect her hands causing shaking and an inability to hold onto the brushes. She told the *Los Angeles Times* that "the impact [MS] had on my art is total." In a video for the *Times's* website, she discussed having to tie her brushes to her hands with laces or bra straps in order to be able to paint. MS also eventually compromised Lydia's vision in one eye, which affected her ability to discern perspective, something vital for artists. In addition to tethering her brushes to her hands, she also wound up wearing an eyepatch.

But by 2021, she invited a documentarian to follow her as she painted what she called her "last mural" because her disabilities had irreversibly progressed to the point where she thought she couldn't paint murals any longer.

In her 2024 memoir, Lydia said she started to use a handicapped placard before her disabilities became visible, which used to earn her "a lot of dirty looks."

But now, coupled with her MS-influenced memory issues, Lydia said the placard has become doubly useful. "It's the best because with my memory loss, it's almost impossible to find my car," she said. "But I can always just look for the blue!"

Seeking Accommodations:
At Work & Public Venues
◆
Noelle
FORMER LICENSED CLINICAL SOCIAL WORKER,
RECREATIONAL BOXER: SECONDARY PROGRESSIVE MS

Noelle was supposed to attend a parents' night at the school where her daughter was a student. However the building was inaccessible to her due to her mobility challenges and MS symptoms.

"I would have to climb up three flights of stairs to get to the third floor to see all of my children's teachers," Noelle explained. "And there's no air conditioning, so if it's a hot and humid night, it is very difficult for me to be there."

The previous year, she described Back to School Night as "a disaster" for her because she thought she could push through those obstacles. Noelle said her attitude was: "You could do it. You're just like everyone else. Yes, you have a kid and you have a walker and you have a placard and you have all these challenges, but you rock it. You rock it every day."

But reality was unkind.

The following year, she realized she needed to ask for accommodations or simply make other arrangements. Her MS, combined with the conditions in the building, were impediments she needed to address.

So after the disaster year, Noelle decided to ask for what she needed. "This year, I feel very proud of myself that … I emailed the teachers and said, 'I am not coming to the open house,'" she said. "The school is not accessible to me. It is not a good situation and what can you do to connect me with the teachers."

Doing this sort of thing has made Noelle uncomfortable. "I'm nervous about being judged for asking for accommodations," she said, "but the only person that's really judging me is me, especially in this situation because I am completely and utterly supported by that school. That's why my kids are at that school because they have really helped my children be able to be supported."

Using her handicap placard out in the world sometimes has felt difficult, even though she now uses a range of mobility devices, which visually answers the questions people have about why someone her age is using a disabled placard.

"Unfortunately, a lot of people in society feel that they have every right to know why I'm using mobility [devices] or why I'm using a handicapped placard," Noelle said. "There's this trying to relate and show empathy, but then the only way that I can explain is by giving my diagnosis and telling strangers. I can't tell you how many strangers on any given day that I have to tell I have MS."

Her advice for those who are newly-diagnosed and in need of accommodations? "Don't be ashamed of it. Advocate. Go for it, you know. But accommodations, it's tough because you're sometimes sticking out like a sore thumb."

She also warned folks who use a mobility aid when their disabilities are invisible it can also be challenging. Noelle related an instance when she and her husband parked in a disabled spot outside of a coffee shop and a woman, who thought Noelle was faking her disability, took a photo of Noelle's license plate. She mustered the courage to confront the woman and inform her that she had MS. "I have a disability," she said. "It is a hidden disability, but it is still a disability and I have every right to use that placard."

Noelle said she has undergone questioning in parking lots from police officers who didn't believe she was actually disabled. One day, she parked in a disabled spot outside an arts and crafts store and decided to use a shopping cart to help support and steady her instead of her walker as she and her children went shopping. When Noelle returned to her vehicle, an officer was waiting for her and proceeded to grill her for over a half hour about why she was parked in a disabled spot, citing the rampant cases of fraudulent placard use.

"Finally, I just looked at him and I told him that I had MS and he kind of had a hard time [believing me]. He's telling me that one of his fellow officers had [MS] and was older and disabled," Noelle said. Ultimately, she showed the officer the placard with her face on it—placards come with privacy shields to cover the owner's face—and said, "Look, this is my placard. This is me. Can I please leave? Can I please go?"

When flying commercial airlines, she said she's experienced similar "disrespect" and "questioning" and was once told that if she couldn't handle physical tasks such as placing her suitcase on a conveyor belt, she had no business traveling alone. Noelle has had her wheelchair disappear from cargo holds and has wound up stuck on a plane because of snafus in getting her assistance with disembarking.

Noelle said one of the ways she faces having to seek accommodations and utilize mobility aids is to make sure they're cool looking and boost her morale.

"If I'm going to be disabled, I'm gonna be stylish," she said. "... I am trying to break the stigma around using mobility aids and show that I am worth it in this world."

Seeking Accommodations:
At Work & Public Venues
◆
Dr. Tanuja Chitnis
NEUROLOGIST SPECIALIZING IN MS AND PEDIATRIC NEUROLOGY

Dr. Chitnis said she and her staff regularly help their pediatric patients with the accommodations they may need for school and other activities.

For children who haven't yet graduated from high school, she and her staff create plans for ADA accommodations, including time off for medical appointments. For those who are college-aged, the Mass General Pediatric MS Clinic staff help not only with obtaining the ADA accommodations, but also with getting a variety of services based on their individual cases of MS.

Dr. Chitnis said clinic staff have written accommodation letters for college students who need ground-level dorm rooms and sometimes even air conditioning. Additionally, they can help students request specialized care in classrooms.

For Dr. Chitnis's adult patients, she said: "If there are symptoms that are starting to affect them in their workplace or in their daily activities, even with mothers and someone who's not working outside the home, if they find that the fatigue is really affecting them, I encourage them to speak with our social worker on accommodations. We have lots and lots of patients who we've sought short-term accommodations for, and even long-term disability."

But for some professions or just because of patient preferences, Dr. Chitnis said some prefer not to make their direct supervisors aware of their MS-related needs. However, there's a way around that, Dr. Chitnis suggested. "If you feel that you can manage and that you have the accommodations you need without telling anyone, then that's fine," she said. "If you do need accommodations, let's say, an air-conditioned office, we can write a letter to take to HR. Your boss doesn't necessarily have to know. Or, if you feel comfortable, you can speak to your boss, your coworkers. We now have more protections in place for people with any diagnosis."

CHAPTER FIVE

Getting the Help You Need:
Tests, Medicines, Treatments & Therapy

Getting the Help You Need:
Tests, Medicines, Treatments & Therapy
◆
Meredith
WRITER, LECTURER, MS ADVOCATE: RELAPSING REMITTING MS

My neurologist and I had exchanged a number of messages via the patient portal. I needed a refill of Ondansetron, the medicine I take for the nausea I experience when in heat and humid conditions. Without it, making it through very hot or very humid days, is very challenging, sometimes impossible. I only take the medicine when conditions on the ground warrant it. I take a lot of it during damp springs and steamy summers, much less when the crispness of New England autumns settle in and the frost curls on the windows. Yet, because of the opaqueness of health insurance, the dictates of pharmacy benefit managers (PBM), obtaining my prescription refills can be an infuriating process. Depending on the whims of the PBMs handling my health insurers' clients, I may be told I can no longer go to my local pharmacy, but instead need to fill the prescription at another drugstore chain. Or they'll only give me nine tablets at a time, not the full month's worth. Trying to use the online portals was fruitless and afforded me ample opportunities to hurl profanity at my laptop, a reaction which frightened my Jack Russell Tedy and, even prompted Scott to pop his head into my office to see if I was okay. (Reader: I was not okay.)

Lucky for me, my neurologist stuck with it and advocated for me to get that medicine. He sent faxes and online messages and made calls. He refiled things he'd already filed because someone in some office somewhere was impersonating a doorstop, standing between me and the medicine I needed to enable me to do my work when the summer weather was making it difficult. (I learned that even when I'm safely inside an air conditioned locale, if the humidity and dew points are high enough, the conditions inside buildings can still ignite my heat sensitivity.)

I wrote my neurologist a note in June 2022, telling him that a customer service rep from my insurance company asked that I ask him to "resubmit the Ondansetron prescription for nine pills at a time. Apparently my insurance doesn't cover more than nine pills per [prescription]. They told me they would not approve coverage until the script is resubmitted."

Less than an hour later (have I mentioned how much I love my current neurologist?), he wrote back: "Oh, the silly games we must play ... nine tabs it is!"

I continue to appreciate his willingness to follow up on all of my prescription needs, even when he fully expects to meet a wall of denials. If he thinks I need it, he is as persistent as my Jack Russell. And, he takes reports of my symptoms seriously. Not all neurologists do. Some pooh-pooh patients' reports, particularly when the symptoms with which they're grappling cannot be objectively measured by the practitioner. My neurologist treats me like a partner in this health care journey, not like I'm a shaking ignoramus who needs to be told to stop worrying so much because he's never heard of the symptoms about which I'm concerned.

To put this in perspective, it's important that you know that I typically avoid interpersonal conflict whenever I'm able whether I'm on the phone or someone is right in front of me. In the realm of medical care, I am irrationally concerned about being labeled a difficult or needy patient. I want the doctors, the physician assistants, the nurses, the techs, the admin staff, the customer service people for the health insurer, and the pharmacist all to think I'm a perfectly pleasant woman, reasonable, and low-maintenance. I am loath to push back or to advocate in ways that might shatter the people-pleasing facade. (Don't mess with my family members, however, in which case I can be ferocious and tenacious.)

Don't be like me.

Push. Advocate. Ask. Demand. Your health, your physical, cognitive, and emotional wellbeing is well worth the price of having someone deciding you're a Karen or a Ken. This is not a game. Your quality of life is worth the effort.

In an April 2024 episode of their podcast MeSsy, actors Jamie-Lynn Sigler and Christina Applegate, who both have MS, discussed how important it was to them to use a wheelchair when they're in an airport even though it made them uncomfortable, to use what they need to make living in their lives possible.

Sigler, who said she walks with a cane, said: "It took me a while to finally ask for it. I felt bad asking for it. I felt weird asking for it, but it is a savior."

Applegate, who'd recently traveled to Europe with her family, agreed saying that as much as she didn't want to use them, airport wheelchairs are "a game changer."

"I don't know if you feel this way when you get into an airport, the anxiety of being in an airport, the lighting, the people, the rush, the energy, affects your nervous system," Applegate added later, " ... [A]ny kind of stress or anxiety will [make me] start to shut down. My legs will just go to noodles and be done."

Push. Advocate. Ask. Demand. You only have this one life. Don't waste it.

Getting the Help You Need:
Tests, Medicines, Treatments & Therapy
◆
Elissa
COMMUNICATIONS & MARKETING DIRECTOR, NOVELIST: RELAPSING REMITTING MS

Elissa said she had a difficult time when she changed health insurers because it disrupted her ability to access specialty MS medication, which cannot be purchased at a corner pharmacy. "There were several months where things did not go smoothly, copay assistance got messed up, I had to pay much higher amounts, and I even had a lapse in the medication while things were figured out," she said, adding that finally getting her medication is often a "constant struggle" involving many messages and calls.

As far as being prescribed much-needed medication, Elissa said she's lucky she has a neurologist who listens to her and tries to give her what she needs. "I was very appreciative when my neurologist was willing to prescribe me Modafinil for fatigue," she said. "It has made a world of difference for me in helping me have increased energy levels, which in turn, helps me to implement healthier habits, like regular exercise, which boosts my energy, strength, and balance."

Her advice for the newly-diagnosed when it comes to getting what they need for their MS? "Keep a list of essential phone numbers, email addresses, and websites handy. Set reminders for when to check in or when deadlines arise. I can say from experience, don't rely on your memory from the prior month! Ask for help when needed from a friend or family members who can help with calls, or at least help keep track of dates and deadlines, if possible."

Getting the Help You Need:
Tests, Medicines, Treatments & Therapy
◆
Sarah
FORMER CUSTOMER SERVICE AND WAREHOUSE SUPERVISOR,
MS SOCIAL MEDIA INFLUENCER AND ADVOCATE: RELAPSING REMITTING MS

Overall, Sarah considers herself fortunate to have been able to get the treatments and medicine she needs even though her family, which used to rely on Medicare and Medi-Cal, now makes too much money for government-subsidized health care.

"I freaked out because losing that meant I was going to have to come up with more money for my copays now," she said. "I'm not that familiar with how the business side of my Medicare works so I reached out online asking for help and I got so many great tips from people on who to talk to and what questions I should ask. The best supplemental plan means I have to pay $8,000 out-of-pocket for my meds before my insurance will pay for it, but it's covered for the rest of [a year], so thankfully, I just have to pay my $4 copay for my DMT."

She said she would be scoping out "different forms of Medicare" for which she might qualify. "I am so thankful that there are people who have gone through similar situations and have tips and tricks to help each other out," she said.

When she was first diagnosed, an emergency room physician told her to ask the neurologist she saw to prescribe Tysabri, a medicine delivered by IV infusion roughly every month, "because my MS was presenting so aggressive."

However, like Elissa, her insurance wouldn't pay for it because it adhered to the step therapy method.

"My insurance would only approve the cheapest medications and made me fail [which led to MS progression] on two of the oldest and not the most effective DMTs before they finally okayed to put me on a 'better' pill, DMT," Sarah said. "Still, not the treatment I was told would be the best for me, and I'm not sure how much money it would actually have saved them because my MS kept progressing and I was still having to go to PT for my leg."

Sarah added that it's important to bring someone with you to be your ears and your advocate when trying to take in all the moving parts and confusing lingo used in the medical system.

"I have a hard time concentrating in doctor appointments with what the doctor is saying," Sarah said. "... It's hard to be our advocates sometimes. I don't always realize I'm walking weird or I forget to bring things up. If you can't be your own advocate, find someone who can. My mom has no issue fighting my doctors for me."

Getting the Help You Need:
Tests, Medicines, Treatments & Therapy
◆
Paige
FORMER IT SYSTEMS ANALYST, FORMER ENDURANCE ATHLETE,
MS SOCIAL MEDIA INFLUENCER: RELAPSING REMITTING MS

Paige has had to employ any number of strategies to get the MS medicine and treatments she needs and always anticipates problems.

"Insurance will almost always deny the DMTs at first," she said. "This happened to me and I later learned from my community that this is normal. Let the doctor's office know and they should take care of it."

Paige said she's struggling to locate a pharmacy that'll fill her prescriptions for specialized medicine.

"Accessing treatment can be a battle sometimes. I have to stay on top of what I need. I've had to take on responsibilities for my own well-being which was difficult for me at first, and still is," she said. "Due to therapies being so expensive, it's been difficult to keep up with it all."

Her speech and language pathologist has provided her with incredible support. "She is someone I could hang out with as a friend," Paige said. "She has gotten to know my 'tells' better than me. I struggle cognitively and she has helped me recognize my 'tells' and what I can do to avoid brain fatigue."

Getting the Help You Need:
Tests, Medicines, Treatments & Therapy
◆
Eddy
SOFTWARE PROFESSIONAL, NATIONAL MS SOCIETY BOARD OF TRUSTEE MEMBER
AND MS ADVOCATE: RELAPSING REMITTING MS

When Eddy's MS journey started "there were very few drugs on the market." He wound up selecting an injectable medication as his disease-modifying medication.

"While new meds have been released, including oral tablets, I have found it difficult to figure out how much it would cost if I changed," he said. "Health insurance plans are not always very clear. I'm also worried that a different drug will not work as well as my current treatment. While I definitely have injection fatigue, weighing the risks/benefits of changing is difficult."

One of the things with which Eddy struggles is getting through MRIs and he's had the support of staff to cope with his anxiety. "I've had techs who suggest placing a towel over my eyes to block my view or offer music during MRIs," he said. "The best techs, however, are those who do not come across as judgmental or frustrated. And anti-anxiety medications do not hurt."

His advice for new MS patients? "Do not be afraid to speak up. And do not feel guilty or bad for having a tough time. They are there to care for you."

Getting the Help You Need:
Tests, Medicines, Treatments & Therapy
◆
Lydia
MURALIST, ARTIST, AUTHOR: PROGRESSIVE MS

In the 2022 documentary *The Art of Rebellion*, about Lydia's art and her MS experience, there was a powerful scene where she clutched a stack of mail, unpaid medical bills, to her chest and lamented what she saw as the intentionally opaque and difficult-to-navigate medical system. A large portion of the documentary addressed Lydia's difficulty trying to pay for her medical care, while simultaneously trying to work, to care for her daughters, and cope with her accumulating MS symptoms.

In a 2015 *Los Angeles Times* video, Lydia was depicted painting a mural promoting U.S. Senator Bernie Sanders's presidential campaign. She told the *Times* that before the passage of the Affordable Care Act in 2010 she couldn't get healthcare. Her art, she said, has always been political and her MS art was the politics of the personal.

Getting the Help You Need:
Tests, Medicines, Treatments & Therapy
◆
Noelle
FORMER LICENSED CLINICAL SOCIAL WORKER,
RECREATIONAL BOXER: SECONDARY PROGRESSIVE MS

Noelle's husband owns a small construction company so her family buys their own private insurance.

"We make too much of an income in order to get any assistance with paying for health insurance," she said, "so health insurance is out-of-pocket for private health insurance and it is very, very expensive. And we've chosen the only way we can kind of do that is by having deductibles, which I, of course, max out pretty fast. But even with paying a private insurance, so much money."

Costs aside, it is a challenge for Noelle to get the numerous prescriptions she needs filled.

"Getting what I need is still jumping through hoops, which is really difficult and frustrating to be living with the chronic illness and dealing with the healthcare system," she said.

In spite of her experience working in hospitals, as a patient it can be infuriating to weave one's way through the thicket that is the healthcare system. "It's still really hard, even if you work through an advocate with the MS Society or with your clinic where you go see your neurologist. Sometimes, it's still not as cut and dried. There's a lot of loopholes. There's a lot of tricky spots."

Getting her mobility aids covered by insurance—especially aids that represent Noelle's desire to boost her self-esteem with their flair—is arduous.

"Nothing is really covered, especially if you want something fancy," Noelle said. "As someone who uses mobility aids on a daily basis, my motto is: 'If I'm going to be disabled, I'm going to … find products that make my self-esteem higher and make me feel good, almost fashionable.' These products, to me, are almost accessories in my life. And it's really hard because they are very, very expensive if you want to look good."

Even aids that aren't fashionable, she said, can be hard for patients to obtain: "Even if you just want a wheelchair, like if I want an electric wheelchair, I would not be covered due to the fact that I am mostly ambulatory, but at any given day, at any given moment, I might be walking in the morning, but then at night time, I can no longer walk. And because I am an ambulatory disabled person who sometimes requires a wheelchair, it is not covered."

She asked the insurance company to cover a scooter but the company said no because she said she's "not able to use the scooter inside my house. That's a silly rule. Who uses a scooter inside a house? Like, scooters are for giving independence outside "in" the world, not inside your house. So it's really expensive, I mean, I've been looking at scooters and they can range to $2,500."

A muscle-stimulating device for her leg that helps her walk changed her life. It was not covered by insurance. "I found out that it wasn't, and that was a devastating blow because the price point was so astronomical that I'm lucky that I have the support around me and different foundations that I'm connected with that were able to help me get the device," Noelle said of the device which straps around her leg.

In order to get her DMT IV infusions every four weeks in her home, she said there were serious obstacles but she eventually overcame them.

"My nurses, who, over the years, I've had two come into my house for the infusion, and they are a force to be reckoned with," Noelle said. "They advocate for me when they see that my blood pressure is low. They fought really hard to be able to get me the extra fluid that they felt that I needed to be safe. They spoke to my doctors when health insurance stuff happened. They, the insurance and CVS, were kind of dragging their feet and I was gonna miss my infusion, which really screws up my cycle and how I feel. And so my nurse actually slipped me the number of an insurance person for me to speak to, and I called and gave the saga of my sad story. You find those people that do go above and beyond to advocate for you to make sure that you get what you need."

Her advice to new patients? "Never stop fighting," she said. "It is hard, but try to find the people who are willing to advocate for you. Your doctor's office, the social worker, even an advocate."

Noelle continued: "I have a really good friend who really found herself in a tough situation and really needed to navigate the system, which was really hard—the insurance system, the disability system—but luckily she was able to find people to help her. And now she has created this amazing website that you can go to and she kind of walks you through disability and different resources for health insurance and the SNAP program, and all that kind of stuff, and I think that that's an amazing resource."

Lastly, she says to keep pushing for your needs because that's what it takes to get things done. "It is really hard, but just keep advocating for yourself to get what you need, to get the resources."

Getting the Help You Need:
Tests, Medicines, Treatments & Therapy
◆
Dr. Tanuja Chitnis
NEUROLOGIST SPECIALIZING IN MS AND PEDIATRIC NEUROLOGY

Dr. Chitnis said she winds up having to advocate with health insurance companies for "about five percent" of her patients.

"We're quite fortunate in Massachusetts, especially with MassHealth [which helps families, seniors and those with disabilities with healthcare and prescriptions] that everyone is covered to some extent," she said. "There are some instances where I have to advocate for the right medicine."

For her pediatric patients, she said getting the right medicine for them can be tricky. "We only have one FDA-approved treatment, Gilenya, which is very good. But there are patients who, for some reason, can't take that or may be suited to another medicine. So, I have to really advocate for other medicines."

Dr. Chitnis said she handles her share of prescription paperwork when prescriptions for medicines and treatments aren't approved by insurance companies. There can be a lot of faxes, she said adding, "And I will say that my office does an amazing job of addressing these challenges and generally, it works out okay."

CHAPTER SIX

Advocating
& Getting Involved with MS Causes

I am only one
But still I am one.
I cannot do everything,
But still I can do something.
And because I cannot do everything
I will not refuse to do the something that I can do.

—Edward Everett Hale

Advocating
& Getting Involved with MS Causes
◆
Meredith
WRITER, LECTURER, MS ADVOCATE: RELAPSING REMITTING MS

In 2017, I outed myself publicly as a person living with MS. The prospect of losing the legal protections preventing health insurers from discriminating against people with preexisting conditions like MS forced my hand.

A little background: I've been obsessed with news and politics since I was an undergraduate at UMass-Amherst, where I earned a BA in journalism and political science. The first piece I had published in the student newspaper, the *Massachusetts Daily Collegian*, was an opinion piece about flag-burning legislation. I loved researching it and writing it. I became staff as a weekly columnist where I tackled myriad political topics of the late 1980s and early 1990s. I transitioned to news reporting and, after becoming the editor-in-chief, graduated and soon became a professional newspaper reporter. A few years later, I wanted to deepen my knowledge of American government, so I obtained my MA in political science while working as an investigative reporter writing about the 1996 presidential race.

Even though I'd go on to write parenting and pop culture columns for several years following the birth of my children, even though I wrote a novel about mommy blogging and a work of creative nonfiction about a middle school jazz band in mourning, I've remained riveted by the American political scene. Back when I was using Twitter (I still have an account but it hasn't been active since 2023 due to issues I have with its owner) you'd find me live-tweeting all manner of political debates, State of the Union addresses, even an insurrection.

So when my fear began to mount in the summer of 2017 as the Republican majorities in the House of Representatives and the U.S. Senate were set to cast votes to repeal many of the provisions of the 2010 Affordable Care Act (ACA), I felt compelled to say something. If the ACA was repealed, those who have or have had illnesses—from cancer, mental health, and heart ailments, to diabetes, asthma, and multiple sclerosis—could be denied health insurance coverage, a practice the Obama-era legislation banned. Should my spouse, through whose company we obtained our health insurance, switch or lose his job, without the ACA protections, insurers could take one look at me, someone who has yearly MRIs, visits a pricey neurologist twice a year, and takes expensive prescription medicine, and say, "No. We're not covering her." Without insurance coverage, my family couldn't afford to pay out-of-pocket for my care. Without my disease-modifying medication and without my neurologist's care, my disease could and likely would worsen, potentially render me unable to continue working.

The campaign to do away with the ACA, led by then-President Donald Trump, felt incredibly personal. On May 6, 2017, I told my thousand-plus followers this on the social media platform formerly known as Twitter:

This Vox column is so powerful #IAmAPreexistingCondition

I didn't give any details about what my pre-existing condition was, only that I had one. This changed two months later as the possibility of the ACA being repealed grew more likely and I publicly revealed my MS diagnosis, tweeting:

Prescription drug coverage is so important to my family.
Without coverage, my MS meds cost over $80K+. Annually.
#iamapreexistingcondition

It took me another year before I began writing for the National MS Society's blog, addressing topics like how legislation could affect MS patients, to my daily life's experiences living with a chronic illness. I shared the posts online, from my Facebook feed to Instagram. The big secret I'd been harboring burst out into the open. By 2020, my MS memoir was published and my employer also knew about my chronic illness.

It seems inevitable now, in retrospect, what happened next, given my interest in politics and in informing people about an illness for which there is so little, genuine understanding. In 2022, I joined the Greater New England Chapter of the MS Society's Board of Trustees, meaning I'd be asked to not only monetarily contribute to the Society, but I'd be expected to raise money as well as awareness. Given my background and interest in news and politics, I soon found myself on the Massachusetts chapter's Government Relations Advisory Committee. I received training and lobbied state and federal officials—in one-on-one meetings, at a public event at the Massachusetts State House, and via online meetings with staff—on bills that would affect the MS community, such as preventing what's called "non-medical switching" (when insurers insist patients switch to a lower-cost drug as opposed to the one prescribed by a physician) and modifications to the Federal Aviation Administration's guidelines for disabled access on new airplanes.

I would've never imagined that I'd find myself sitting in a meeting room in the Worcester office of U.S. Rep. Jim McGovern, the ranking Democratic member on the House Committee on Rules soon after he'd been profiled in *The New Yorker,* discussing with him the impact of pharmacy benefit managers (PBMs) on people trying to obtain necessary medication. I got to detail for Rep. McGovern how difficult it was for me to obtain my anti-nausea medication. It enabled me to endure heat and humidity without becoming listless, unfocused, dizzy or sick to my stomach. And while there is no cure for my MS, no magic solution to *poof* enable me to enjoy summers again, I could speak with this elected representative about getting people the help they need, about how legislation and policies could help those with chronic illnesses. I never would've imagined walking the halls of the Massachusetts State House on State Action Day and speaking with my state representative about PBM reform and non-medical switching, nor accompanying another MS Activist, to meet with my state senator in his Marlborough office to discuss those same issues.

At the Unitarian Universalist church I attend in Westborough, Massachusetts, I remember seeing a quote on the Orders of Service from Edward Everett Hale: "I am only one, but still I am one. I cannot do everything, but still I can do something. And because I cannot do everything I will not refuse to do the something that I can do." Whenever the sermon tackled racial discrimination, attacks on LGBTQ rights, or wars in Iraq, Afghanistan, or Gaza, the one thing those of us sitting in the over 150-year-old pews were encouraged to do was to do what we could to help others, to help the world, even if it was something small. I thought of those sermons, of that omnipresent quote that appeared on the printed Orders of Service when I considered what I could contribute to the MS Society. In spite of the limitations placed on me by my MS—the fatigue, the heat sensitivity, and so on—I decided to be selective about how I spend my energy. Speaking to legislators about public policy issues, that was something I could fit into my schedule and could accomplish because of my passion for politics.

And while there are some who, in spite of their MS, can participate in vigorous outdoor events like MS bike rides, marathon runs, etc., I'm not one of them. But I was able to promote the Bike MS team my husband and two sons put together for an event in Maine. They did the physical effort, the biking, the training, and the fundraising by asking people to contribute, so I used my social media presence to spread the word as well. When they rode for the past few years, I sent them love and affection via video chats.

In the spring of 2024, MS Society organizers invited me to "host" two Walk MS events, one in central Massachusetts and one in the western part of Massachusetts. This entailed me writing a short speech about my MS experience and my involvement with the MS Society; a staffer inserted it into a script which I read at each event. The one in central Massachusetts was in Worcester, about twenty minutes from my house, so getting there and back wasn't physically taxing for me. The weather was lovely and delivering the speech thanking participants for raising money to help find a cure and better treatments for multiple sclerosis, as well as spotlighting a team's story, was an honor. The second Walk MS event in Longmeadow—close to where I grew up—was about an hour-and-a-half drive each way and, given that I had to leave early in the morning, Scott kindly served as my driver, enabling me to give the speech and stay on my feet during the bulk of the event as I mingled with participants. Though there were snafus with the handheld microphones and I was thoroughly exhausted when I got home from the events, I was pleased to have been able to pitch in. It made me feel as though I was not just helping others, but was role-modeling what *can* be done even while living with this disease.

As I mentioned in a prior chapter, if I were starting this MS journey over again, I'd reach out to and engage with the MS

Society sooner than I did. I'd try to use my voice and my story to help people understand the disease, even if I just reached a single person.

Advocating
& Getting Involved with MS Causes
◆
Elissa
COMMUNICATIONS & MARKETING DIRECTOR, NOVELIST: RELAPSING REMITTING MS

In the past, Elissa has participated in and co-organized charity walk events for the National MS Society. When the Society stopped hosting Walk MS events in her area, she designed her own, a three-mile charity walk for herself and her family. She also makes sure to support and publicly share fundraising links for other people's MS fundraising efforts.

As a writer, Elissa has raised awareness about multiple sclerosis in other ways. Her first novel, *The Speed of Light*, features a young main character in the first year following her MS diagnosis. "Her journey going through an MS diagnosis, with all the fears and uncertainties, is based on my own," she said.

She also wrote for the National MS Society's blog about her experiences as a young mother with MS and has shared her own personal stories on social media during MS Awareness Week in March and on World MS Day in May.

While her advocacy for and awareness-raising about multiple sclerosis ranges from fundraising to novel writing and blog posting, Elissa said that for newly-diagnosed patients, they need to decide what feels right for them.

"Be as involved as you are able to be," she said. "If you don't want to be in the public eye, that's okay. Maybe you'd prefer to share other people's social media posts or make a donation to a fundraiser rather than attend. Or it's okay if you want nothing to do with it, especially right away. It might change over time, and you might feel more comfortable getting involved later on, so just do whatever you need to do for you."

Advocating
& Getting Involved with MS Causes
◆
Dianne
FORMER LIBRARY AIDE,
MS SUPPORT GROUP CO-LEADER: RELAPSING REMITTING MS

In addition to helping to co-lead her local MS support group, Dianne works hard to raise MS awareness and to educate the public in other ways.

For five years, she served as a patient ambassador for the pharmaceutical company Biogen, which makes several MS drugs, where she "spoke to thousands of people with MS and their caregivers" about her MS journey and the medicine she was taking, fielding questions about her experience with DMTs.

Online, Dianne posts information on Instagram about MS for an MS-centric audience. "I manage my MS-related content on a separate Instagram account from my personal Instagram account, not because I'm ashamed of MS, but because it allows me to stay more connected with the MS community in a focused way, without mixing it with my everyday life on my main account." Her posts range from positive-thinking memes, such as "Tough times never last but tough people do," to posts about bladder incontinence MS symptoms.

To patients who are early in their journey, she is encouraging.

"Share your story," Dianne said. "Your personal journey with MS and the profound impact it has had on your life holds significant advocacy potential. Your story can inspire others and raise awareness about the realities of living with MS."

Advocating
& Getting Involved with MS Causes
◆
Sarah

FORMER CUSTOMER SERVICE AND WAREHOUSE SUPERVISOR,
MS SOCIAL MEDIA INFLUENCER AND ADVOCATE: RELAPSING REMITTING MS

Six years after she was diagnosed with MS—soon after she experienced a "horrible relapse" that twice landed her in the hospital and after she learned the disease had spread to her spine—Sarah said she had a "heart-to-heart" with MS "about us living together" and decided, since her MS wasn't going anywhere, she would get involved in advocating on behalf of MS causes.

Speaking out about multiple sclerosis was intimidating at first. "I almost always get imposter syndrome, because why would anyone want to talk to me?" Sarah said. "... Sharing my story has really helped me find my voice."

She has been deeply involved with the MS Society by appearing in educational videos and lobbying state and federal officials as a District Activist Leader on subjects relevant to MS patients. She speaks with state officials in California's capital of Sacramento, and with her state's members of Congress in Washington, D.C. As a member of her local MS chapter's Government Relations Board, Sarah also helps determine the policies for which they'll lobby: issues that are vital to the MS community.

Sarah also spends a lot of time online raising public awareness about the disease so, when the next person gets diagnosed, the public may be a bit more knowledgeable.

"I post to my social media whenever I think of something to share," Sarah said. "I write random blog posts and am occasionally recognized at MS events, which is funny to me. I have worked with a few MS patients' websites to give my answers on surveys or to discuss living with MS. I use the term 'living with MS' instead of saying I have MS because, for me, it is something that lives with me."

To new patients, she said, "It's your story. I encourage people to share what they are comfortable with. Maybe that's being an open book or maybe that's lurking on social media and just finding information on creators' accounts."

Advocating
& Getting Involved with MS Causes
◆
Paige

FORMER IT SYSTEMS ANALYST, FORMER ENDURANCE ATHLETE,
MS SOCIAL MEDIA INFLUENCER: RELAPSING REMITTING MS

Over twenty-thousand people benefit from Paige's TikTok videos—which she posts under the name MS Fighter 101—explaining all aspects of multiple sclerosis, sometimes while she's deftly applying makeup and speaking into the camera.

"I started posting videos in an effort to help others learn and understand MS," she said. "The anxiety and stress I was under in 2018 when everything started, I wanted to help others get through that not feeling alone. My goal has always been to help others."

Paige has also served as a patient ambassador for the website, myMSteam, a venture-capital-backed startup group of sites called MyHealth Team, through which MS patients can seek support.

Her advice for new MS patients: "It's a personal choice of how active you want to be about sharing your story and advocating. Getting involved with raising awareness can be exhausting and having a chronic, progressive condition makes it one hundred times harder."

Advocating
& Getting Involved with MS Causes

◆

Eddy

SOFTWARE PROFESSIONAL, NATIONAL MS SOCIETY BOARD OF TRUSTEE MEMBER
AND MS ADVOCATE: RELAPSING REMITTING MS

Eddy, who is on the National MS Society's Greater New England Board of Trustees and oversees community engagement for this chapter, said he first became involved in advocacy "because a friend with MS reached out and said we needed to be a part of the MS Society."

Not only does his involvement as a volunteer enable him to connect with other MS patients, but it empowers him to advocate for something that personally affects his life. "In addition, it keeps me close to the source of important information, where are we with research, treatment, cure, etc."

He added, "I find some purpose in talking with those diagnosed with MS who are looking to talk to someone and maybe find some hope."

For those new to MS, Eddy said: "Any little bit helps the cause, as well as you. Even participating in [an MS walk] will open your eyes to a great community. Getting more deeply involved can also keep you connected and provide sources of information that can help you throughout your journey."

Advocating
& Getting Involved with MS Causes
◆
Lydia
MURALIST, ARTIST, AUTHOR: PROGRESSIVE MS

Working with the MS Society in the mid-2010s, Lydia created a series of "End MS Forever" murals in Los Angeles, Portland, Houston, and Louisville in which she said she "tried to use images of movement." The murals pop with color and depict women in flowy clothing and prominently feature vivid flowers. For example, one of Lydia's most prominent murals appears on the side of a tall Los Angeles building, featuring a woman with a wavy, watermelon-pink dress and a crown of white and yellow flowers atop her wavy, dark brown hair. The woman appears to float on a river of blossoms that starts on a low wall and ends at the bottom of the tall wall. Above those blossoms, in black and white are the words "End Multiple Sclerosis Forever." Encircling the woman's head and torso is a white ring—almost halo-like—which, in pink lettering promises, "There is always hope."

In December 2015, Lydia told the *Los Angeles Times*: "I know my time is short. So my work is about: What can I do in that time, how can I help? What kind of example can I be for my girls? I can't sing. I can't write, but I can paint. This is something I can do."

Lydia also became a face of resilience in a series of videos and appearances on behalf of the MS Society.

Advocating
& Getting Involved with MS Causes
◆
Noelle
FORMER LICENSED CLINICAL SOCIAL WORKER,
RECREATIONAL BOXER: SECONDARY PROGRESSIVE MS

Noelle's perspective as someone who developed MS as a teen gives her a different message to deliver.

"Right now, my crossroads is really trying to be an advocate. All I want to do is help others and break this societal stigma against young adults or ... people living in their 40s using mobility devices or assistive aids," Noelle said. "I just want to break that stigma. Yes, I'm 42, but I am rocking it, using a cane, using a walker, using technology."

She wants to role-model flourishing in her life with MS. "For me, it's about a rocking attitude. There are challenges and I don't deny that living with a chronic illness [is] challenging, but I feel that all my challenges have made me stronger, more determined, more caring, and empathetic for others."

Early in her MS journey, she served on an MS Society advisory committee for young adults and helped organize activities and educational programs, as well as spoke to newly-diagnosed young people. During that time, she and her family also became very involved in raising money for MS walks, but she's since scaled back those efforts in favor of using social media to "talk about the challenge of MS and also to try to give a safe space to be able to talk about the tough stuff, not just the wonderful times."

Noelle also currently helps her local chapter of the MS Society with a fashion show fundraiser featuring women with MS, including her, as the runway models.

"I'm part of the MS Society on the Fashion Plates Committee every year, and that's what I feel is really important to me, spreading awareness about chronic illness, spreading awareness about MS, raising money, and really trying to push back against society, [to say] I am just as important as anyone else."

Noelle dons the clothing and uses her mobility aids on the runway. She wants to deliver an incontrovertible message about MS patients: "We are still people. We still matter. And this feeling that we get, or I get, that I'm lesser of some sort because I use [mobility aids] or others feel bad for me. Don't feel bad for me. Be inspired. See what I can do, not what I can't do."

Advocating
& Getting Involved with MS Causes
◆
Laura
ASSISTANT VICE PRESIDENT FOR STATE ADVOCACY AND
POLICE FOR THE NATIONAL MS SOCIETY

Laura has been a professional lobbyist and advocate for a variety of nonprofit organizations, including health-related organizations for patients with cancer, heart disease, and since 2018, multiple sclerosis with the National Multiple Sclerosis Society. She has been the associate vice president of state advocacy and policy for the MS Society since August 2023. Her role is to help support state advocacy staff and volunteers in analyzing legislation and prioritizing public policy issues to support in their states, chapters, and professional staff to help determine on which public policy issues their government advocacy volunteers should direct their efforts.

"Our advocacy work is centered around the needs of people affected by MS and it involves us asking a lot of questions and then taking action," Laura said. "What issues are they facing and how can we address those issues? What would legislation look like and does it exist or do we need to help in developing it? Who in the legislature can we get to be our champion on the issue? How can we best share the experiences of people living with MS to demonstrate the need for change?"

She and other professional advocates at the Society examine existing policies, laws, and proposals to see how they're affecting MS patients, and identify areas of need that remain unaddressed.

"As we identify legislation, we also empower people affected by MS to share their stories related to those policy issues in an effort to motivate lawmakers to act," Laura said.

Between 2023 through September 2024, Laura said the National MS Society held 24 State Action Days across the United States where volunteers (*Disclosure: I volunteered in Massachusetts.*) lobbied their state lawmakers about policies relevant to the MS community. In March 2024, 170 volunteer MS Activists gathered in Washington, D.C. for the National MS Society's Public Policy Conference and then lobbied members of Congress for the expansion of telehealth services and funding MS research through the U.S. Department of Defense.

An MS Activist, Laura explained, is the name the Society gives to its volunteer policy advocates, most of whom live with MS, have a loved one with MS, or are medical professionals who care for MS patients. "These MS Activists take on a number of roles from emailing their elected officials to testifying before elected officials and everything in between," Laura said. "We work to find the best fit for each individual based on their time commitment, level of comfort and areas of interest."

The activists can work on a state level to influence state-based policies and legislation by speaking with state lawmakers, or on federal policies and legislation by speaking directly with members of Congress either in the U.S. Capitol or in their district offices in their home states.

Why does the MS Society utilize the services of MS Activists instead of just relying on paid, professional lobbyists? "Staff can bring facts and figures to an office and have absolutely no impact," Laura said, "but if we bring a real person who has a compelling story? That makes a difference. Those stories stick with you long after you've heard them and legislators and their staff remember those people as they go to cast a vote. Often, the elected officials have no idea of the real-life impact until they hear it directly from someone struggling. They can understand that the cost of MS medications is high with the charts and graphs we provide, but they can't understand that someone is forced to choose between medication and food or rent until they hear that story. The power of stories means everything."

However, Laura said the process of modifying and passing legislation can take several years and go through repeated starts and stops. For example, it took a decade to get a bill passed in Massachusetts to reform "step therapy," where insurance companies didn't cover the medicine an MS patient's doctor prescribed but required the patient to try and fail on cheaper medicines placed lower on an insurer's list of covered prescription medication—called a drug formulary—and if they didn't help the patient, try the next one, and the next one. Only after a patient failed on the drug (or drugs) or went through the required "steps" were they able to access their doctor-prescribed medication. However, during that time when the medicines don't work for the patients, their disease can progress and the symptoms they experience can possibly become permanent. Passage of the step therapy reform bill in 2022 "involved a lot of meetings with legislators, discussions with other patient advocacy groups about the best plan of action each step of the way, calls from MS Activists to legislative offices, and visits to members at the [Massachusetts] State House," Laura said.

She has worked with MS Activists who've testified before legislative committees to tell their stories about their lives with MS and how laws and policies affect them. In one Connecticut case, an MS Activist's testimony about health insurers who, in the middle of a health plan year, changed the list of medicines they'd cover—leading to huge out-of-pocket expenses for patients whose medications are some of the most expensive in the United States—remained lodged in a committee chairperson's mind. Even though it took a few years for it to be reintroduced over and over, that activist's testimony resonated.

"As the bill was debated on the Senate floor, that same committee chair we'd spoken to two years earlier stood up in support of the bill, reading part of an MS Activist's testimony to the rest of the senators," Laura said. "After passage, he took a photo of himself with the vote counter and proudly posted about the new law to social media to share with his constituents."

CHAPTER SEVEN

Living with It

"Sometimes you just have to sit back and look at yourself and what you're doing and just be like, 'But I'm doing it. I'm trying.' And that's so much better than another alternative."

– Jamie-Lynn Siegler, MeSsy Podcast

Living with It

◆

Meredith

WRITER, LECTURER, MS ADVOCATE: RELAPSING REMITTING MS

I had a hankering for a lobster roll. When I emerged from the Harwich Port house and set foot onto the freshly-cut grass in a late summer afternoon, I was thrilled to discover that the hot and muggy Cape Cod weather had faded to the point where I could actually enjoy some time outdoors for a change. My husband Scott and I were sitting on the soft sands of Bank Street Beach at nearly 6 p.m. on a Sunday, the humid breeze cooling our wet bodies ever-so-slightly, when I looked up from my delicious beach read and announced I wanted a lobster roll.

Since I have a dairy allergy, finding one that I can eat safely can be a challenge. While I can have mayonnaise—too many folks make the mistake of thinking that the eggs in mayo are dairy products even though they come from chickens, not cows—I cannot have lobster meat that's been bathed, boiled, or steamed in butter, nor can I have buttery rolls like a brioche that many New England eateries use as the medium on which they serve their famous rolls.

We opted to go to the Dockside Seafood Shack whose ample outdoor seating overlooks the Saquatucket Municipal Marina which leads to the south-facing Nantucket Sound. The kindly proprietor—who had a rack of his daughter's friendship bracelets for sale on the counter and acknowledged that he, himself, is a Swiftie—told me my best bet was to have a Lobster Glow Bowl, not a traditional lobster roll. The bowl featured a generous amount of cold lobster meat served over spinach, quinoa, smoked chickpeas, dried cranberries, and their "signature" dressing, which I was assured was dairy-free. A local teen wearing a Dockside tee and shorts delivered our food on hard blue plastic trays covered by red and white-checked paper. My salad looked so tantalizing that I took a photo of it in all its glossy glory. It would be my first one of the season.

Then I took a bite. And it tasted like nothing.

The taste that lived in my memory—that briny, salty, tang of smooth lobster meat bearing a coat of mayo—remained in my memory, in the past. The Dockside lobster I'd had a year or so ago, laid atop a bed of greens, while not the traditional mayo-covered lobster roll, still had pizazz. But I'm sure it wasn't the food that lacked taste. It was me. And my MS. To my husband, it tasted fine.

MS had stolen something else from me.

Years ago, I noticed that my sense of taste seemed blunted. It reminded me of the same diminished sense of touch I have on the left side of my body thanks to my relapsing remitting multiple sclerosis. Called hypoesthesia, my left-sided numbness is like wearing an invisible layer of fabric, like tights, all the time that obscures my ability to feel what touches my bare skin. On my tongue, not only is my ability to feel the food dulled, but my ability to enjoy the dance of myriad flavors and textures among my tastebuds has been flattened, smothered like a candle snuffer over a flame. It started when I had trouble tasting the salt on Ritz crackers. Then coffee began to taste off, strange, burnt almost, which is a major calamity as I drink at least two cups of coffee each morning. Quickly upon java's heels, red wine—one of my favorite Zinfandels, 7 Deadly Zins—began tasting acidic, even though it wasn't, as Scott confirmed for me.

It's not just me, even though my neurologist at the time said he'd never heard of such a thing and dismissed it. Studies have revealed a correlation between MS and taste dysfunction, including a 2019 paper in the *Community Dentistry and Oral Epidemiology* which found forty percent of those MS patients surveyed indicated experiencing a change in taste, while a 2016 paper in the *Journal of Neurology* found that between fifteen to thirty-two percent experienced taste issues.

In a National MS Society story—for which I was interviewed—a former professional chef with a "classically trained palate," Trevis Gleason said the interruption of one's natural ability to discern tastes is unmooring. He told the magazine *Momentum* that his inability to taste salt was like removing blue from the rainbow. "Blue isn't just sky blue," he said. "If blue isn't there, it makes leaves yellow and the sea black."

So how do I cope with all this, other than getting ticked off and buying loads of taste-packed sauces that I can slather over my food? I'll get back to you on that, as I've not yet made peace with this aspect of my disease. I'm still trying to come up with ways to manage and accept my heat and humidity intolerance in the summers, when my family and friends are able to go to the beach while I'm under house arrest in the air conditioning.

I've saved this hardest topic for the end of this guide. To be honest, I don't think I have a true answer for you, dear reader. As I write this, I've just passed my ten-year anniversary of living with MS and haven't figured this one out yet, how to live with it.

My 2017 memoir *Uncomfortably Numb* ended with a book launch party, at the celebration of a book I feared MS wouldn't allow me to finish. (Clearly I was wrong about that because here I am, still writing, a decade later.) Being able to celebrate the completion and publication of my book, *Mr. Clark's Big Band*, to have been able to make it through that event without a flare-up or fainting or any other physical symptom cropping up (something about which I was having nightmares at the time), to be surrounded by friends who organized and threw the party, to be with people who understood, emotionally buoyed me in a way I hadn't anticipated. It gave me hope that, no matter what avenues or detours my course of MS took, I could handle it.

"I do not fumble my speech," I wrote about the book celebration. "... I do not slur my words. I do not faint. My knees do not buckle. No one has to pick me up off of the floor because I am flying. I do not need to rely on the written speech; I already know it in my heart."

After the jazz band and its alums finished performing a few tunes, their band director, Mr. Clark, dragged me in front of them as the crowd applauded:

"Momentarily horrified and stunned, I am a bashful schoolgirl standing there, uncertain about what I should do with my hands," I wrote. "Members of the crowd rise to their feet. A standing ovation. I've never had one of those before. [Mr. Clark], in his bright cornflower blue shirt which contrasts with my black dress, extends his arms and moves in for a bear-hug. I hug him back and allow the warmth of everything to sink in, down to my bones. In this moment, I am not afraid of the warmth. It is sustaining me. *I'm going to be okay.*"

I'd say that since then, I've been pretty okay, on balance. I've had to reorganize my life around my MS. I need to carefully calibrate where and how I'm going to spend my precious energy, as multiple sclerosis saps most of it pretty quickly.

Our summers are different. Instead of hemming and hawing about whether I can attend an event that will be mostly outdoors, if there isn't an air conditioned area to which I can retreat, I'll just decline the invitation. It's better than having me go, get sick, and then have everyone fuss over me, as I hate the spectacle that can come with MS. It's also preferable to everyone trying to figure out, on the spot, how to deal with me. It also frees my family and friends from worrying and taking care of me so they can instead enjoy themselves. Caring for someone with MS can be as all-encompassing as living with it, so there are times when I just tell Scott to go without me so he can have a moment of mirth without fear. It's why I also don't accompany Scott and my sons to Maine when they participate in a two-day Bike MS event. If I were there, what they can do and where they can go is compromised, so I just take a pass.

I've also learned the lessons Lydia Emily shared: Don't put things off. You need to take advantage of the health and time you have when you have it. In spite of a rather horrifying 2024—Scott had a heart attack, I had a cardiac issue requiring hospitalization, and our beloved 14-year-old mutt Max died in our arms—we decided to move ahead with our plans for a trip to Ireland. Scott was healthy, yet had a genetic abnormality that blocked an artery. I'd never had heart problems yet an errant electrical current landed me on an emergency heart catheterization table. We needed to go to Dublin and Galway in spite of everything because we didn't know what the future holds. We managed my fatigue pretty well, except I became run down and contracted another bad case of COVID. At least we can now say I've set foot on the Emerald Isle.

Living with MS has also meant that I have scaled back on the holidays. We still put out more than enough food (I like leftovers, particularly after I've been expending energy getting ready for a holiday), but it's not all homemade, which would've come as a terrible disappointment to my mother, her mother, and her mother before her, as well as to my late mother-in-law who always took care to ask if my baked goods were from a box or from scratch. Sometimes none of the food is homemade and our biggest challenges are how to reheat everything at the same time. I don't go nuts and scour the house the way I used to in preparation for the holidays, before the MS. Only recently did I give myself permission to pay folks to clean my house twice a month. I'd been spending way too much time beating myself up for not being able to keep the house clean while I was working the equivalent of full-time hours, as was Scott, and my younger son who was living with us. The money spent on cleaning is a gift I gave to myself. If I didn't have MS, I tell myself, I'd be able to clean. But I do have it, and I can't do everything.

This isn't to say that I don't get angry, frustrated, or fed up with the restraints MS places upon me. I do. Often.

I still long for the time when I had boundless energy, or at least I could power myself through my days with massive amounts of caffeine and I needed much less sleep than I do now. I have had to stop measuring my output on any given day and using it to assess whether I've had productive waking hours. This has been a major challenge for me as I pine for when I could plow through my work, still go out grocery shopping (as opposed to getting groceries delivered), make dinner, and do more work (writing, grading) on the other end of my day. I covet those before times when I used to be able to cross out dozens upon dozens of things on my To Do list. This isn't healthy behavior for an MS patient, I know. The memoir I wrote about my first years with multiple sclerosis is divided into two sections, before and after. I live in the "after," as in, after my diagnosis. Meredith with MS is not the same as the Meredith without it. And while that irritates the crap out of me, it's reality.

During one rough patch of time when I was really down about what I perceived as my reduced capacity to complete tasks as compared to what I did before I had MS, my therapist told me to practice something she called "radical acceptance." She meant that I had to extend to myself the same kind of acceptance I would extend to anyone else in my life if they had an illness whose symptoms included the ones with which I live. She urged me to radically accept wherever my body is at any given moment in time, note that, and move on, without judgment. I liked the phrase so much that I wrote it in all caps on a bright green index card and placed it on my desk.

In a June 2024 episode of their MeSsy podcast, Jamie-Lynn Sigler consoled her co-host Christina Applegate who was only a few years into her MS journey compared to Sigler's two decades. Applegate was struggling with the things MS had taken from her life, how MS had shattered her sense of self.

Sigler urged Applegate to focus on what she can do, as opposed to what she can't.

"... [W]hat makes it harder is when you compare [your MS body] to how it used to be," Sigler said. Accepting "this is how it's going to be, maybe forever" is no easy assignment.

In one of their first podcasts together in April 2024, Applegate confessed: "I oftentimes—ninety percent of the time—don't look at the positive side of all of it. I look at the negative side and get bummed out and self-loathing and all of those things, and pissed off, and resentful."

A few weeks later, Sigler encouraged Applegate to give herself time to grieve what MS had taken. "You owe it to yourself to cry and really, really go there," she said. "... You've got to allow yourself to feel that stuff."

Living with It

◆

Elissa

COMMUNICATIONS & MARKETING DIRECTOR, NOVELIST: RELAPSING REMITTING MS

Elissa has lived with MS for over a decade and still has days when she can't stop thinking about it.

"To be honest, daily life is so busy with family and work obligations, so as long as I'm feeling good, I'm usually able to not think about it," she said. "But sometimes I can't push it aside and I worry about the future. When that happens, I talk to my husband, family, or friends, say a prayer, and remind myself that I'm doing all I can to be as healthy as possible for as long as I can."

Sometimes, Elissa revels in a sense of pride about how she's handled it all, how she has plans and back-up plans. Other times, she can experience discouragement where she might think, "No matter what I do, I'm still going to have MS and likely continue to see my health decline. But overall, no matter what, I'm still me. MS might be a part of me, but it's not all of me. And I'm proud and grateful for who I am."

Having an incurable disease has definitely affected how she lives her life and sees her future.

"Sometimes I feel like I fluctuate between trying to plan for the future and take extra care of myself so I can stay healthy as long as possible and feeling like I should live in the moment because tomorrow isn't guaranteed," Elissa said. She tries to strike a balance between the two attitudes making sure she doesn't "put off dreams and goals for some far-off future, and spend time with my kids, family, and friends whenever I can, whether it's planning a trip to Disney, or taking the day off to go to a baseball game."

The uncertainty of her future was a motivating factor for her to complete her first novel. "Now I'm a published author," she said. "No day but today!"

What does she want newly-diagnosed folks to know about the challenge of living with MS? "You are stronger than you think you are," Elissa said. "Every time you think you can't adjust to a new normal, know that you actually can. But don't think that you have to be strong or inspirational all the time. It's okay to feel what you're feeling, to just do your best and live your life."

Living with It

♦

Dianne
FORMER LIBRARY AIDE,
MS SUPPORT GROUP CO-LEADER: RELAPSING REMITTING MS

Dianne says she lives with the uncertainty of her MS by likening MS to her baby.

"Like a parent, I have learned to be adaptable and ready for anything," she said. "There is a constant need for attention and care that MS demands, with unexpected moments that require immediate response. I prioritize tasks and activities based on my energy level and limitations. I appreciate the simple moments of progress and accomplishment because there's immense joy in the small victories. I take care of my MS because it's part of me."

Like Elissa, Dianne said her attitude toward life has shifted since her diagnosis.

"I am more aware of what I can and can't do and that has made me prioritize what is important to me," she said. "I don't want to waste my time and energy. I want to make every moment count."

On the days when she's struggling, Dianne said, "I try to find something positive to be grateful for. I like the practice of 'Three Good Things' which is a mindfulness exercise where you try to think of three good things in your day. It helps me refocus on the good and stop spiraling when I'm feeling bad. Positivity is a choice."

When she suspects a flare of her MS symptoms is about to occur, she informs her people and immediately seeks the help she needs.

"I try to identify and address the trigger," Dianne said. "For example, if I am overheated, I try to cool myself down, both externally and internally, by relocating to a more cooled environment, resting and drinking something really cold."

Her advice: "Multiple sclerosis does not define who you are, but your attitude toward it can shape your journey. Stay positive and know you are not alone."

Living with It

◆

Sarah

FORMER CUSTOMER SERVICE AND WAREHOUSE SUPERVISOR,
MS SOCIAL MEDIA INFLUENCER AND ADVOCATE: RELAPSING REMITTING MS

While she described herself as "pretty chill" before MS came into her life, Sarah said she now thinks hard and plans ahead to decide those activities on which she should expend her finite energy. "That includes both physical and mental energy," she said. "I tend to do my important tasks first thing in the morning because I know my leg is going to start tapping out after lunch. I also try to be present in the moment."

Sarah schedules doctors' appointments for Mondays or Tuesdays because "by Thursday, I am struggling to make it through the week to get my kids to school."

Due to her illness, she said she's learned "to slow down and give myself grace," something she didn't always do before MS.

To new MS patients she says this: "Find ways to make your life easier and don't apologize for it. When I was in the hospital in 2012, my aunt came to sit with me and told me that when people offer to help me, to let them because it makes them feel good and saves you energy if they bring you dinner or grab your dog food while they're out."

Sarah also said she seeks other ways to make life easier.

"I hate to cook, so in the summer, we order from a meal service," she said. "We have also just enacted, 'Fend For Yourself Friday' which means everyone makes their own dinner. It helps us clean out the fridge and freezer to use up food but for me, by Friday, I don't care if we eat toast for dinner because I'm so exhausted by the end of the week."

Living with It

◆

Paige

FORMER IT SYSTEMS ANALYST, FORMER ENDURANCE ATHLETE,
MS SOCIAL MEDIA INFLUENCER: RELAPSING REMITTING MS

Paige said she continues to work on coming to terms with how having this disease has shifted how she sees herself.

"I'm still struggling," she said. "It's been very hard for me to not see myself as the strong, bad-ass triathlete I was, and see myself as chronically ill and disabled."

Since being diagnosed with MS, Paige said, "I try really hard not to focus so much on the future. I live for today and that's it." That means "everything is penciled in, nothing is set in stone, even tomorrow." For someone who previously planned her life out, she said she's trying to embrace being spontaneous.

However, in spite of how MS changes patients' lives, Paige said newly-diagnosed people should know, "This is not the end of the world, but this might rock your world. Listen to your body and always advocate for yourself, and, most importantly, keep moving."

Living with It

◆

Eddy

SOFTWARE PROFESSIONAL, NATIONAL MS SOCIETY BOARD OF TRUSTEE MEMBER
AND MS ADVOCATE: RELAPSING REMITTING MS

Even though Eddy said his MS symptoms are relatively mild, he still frets. "I fluctuate between trying to keep it out of my mind, and then worrying that I will be severely disabled as I age," he said. "Of course, my regular injection is a constant reminder."

He tries to be circumspect about life with a chronic illness. "This may not be the best approach, but I keep in mind that nothing is guaranteed," Eddy said. "Even if I did not have MS, I could not predict what would happen. I suppose I can try to downplay MS because I am fortunate not to have severe symptoms. I realize this is not the same situation for many people with MS and my own situation could change at any time."

Knowing that his MS could worsen prompts him to be aggressive with his physical activity: "I sometimes push myself more because I fear losing physical abilities someday. For example, I may be more motivated not to skip a day at the gym because staying in shape might ward off some MS effects. I'm also more apt to do things because I still can."

Like the other MS patients in this chapter, Eddy said his focus is on the present: "I live a full life that keeps me as engaged and active as I want to be. I remind myself that there are many other things in this life that can be worse than my situation."

Living with It

◆

Lydia

MURALIST, ARTIST, AUTHOR: PROGRESSIVE MS

In a December 2015 *Los Angeles Times* article, Lydia said of her MS: "It's a gift. I would think time is limitless if I wasn't sick. I savor everything now."

She said she copes with the uncertainty of each day by surrounding herself with "the best people possible" for whom she goes "out of my way to do what little things I can for them, and in return, they are like my handlers, as if I was a celebrity."

Her crew would encase her in bubble wrap if they could, Lydia said.

Her days are now organized around her energy and weather conditions.

"I always make sure that I'm never planning to do anything on a hot day," she said. "That is number one! I also avoid stress at all costs." That means using whatever mobility devices she needs including a cane and a wheelchair.

Now that she's stopped painting murals, Lydia says the disease has thoroughly changed how she lives her life, from where she goes to what she eats because she said the disease has led to her developing irritable bowel syndrome. "It's total. Everything."

On difficult days, she said she retreats into "historical, factual dramas and hug my family members." She rests in a cool room and utilizes "lots of pain meds."

Lydia has this advice to new MSers about using time wisely: "If you're newly-diagnosed, do every last thing you possibly can with what you have left. Multiple sclerosis can be like ALS in slow motion. The abilities you have could possibly be slowly taken away. So climb that mountain, run that race, sing that song. Have sex with all your exes, travel the world. Anything that you've ever wanted to do, do with the idea that this could be one of your last chances. And hope that it's not."

Living with It

◆

Noelle

FORMER LICENSED CLINICAL SOCIAL WORKER,
RECREATIONAL BOXER: SECONDARY PROGRESSIVE MS

"I still make a difference and I'm still valued," Noelle said. "I don't know what my future holds, day-to-day, minute-to-minute. It changes, but in my heart, I know that no matter what, I am going to be out in that world, showing people that the stigma around disabilities, chronic illnesses, and ability, and age, needs to change."

She said she never imagined this would be her fate, that she would ever be in a situation where her walking ability is compromised. "And there is grief, even after twenty-some years, that does pop up here and there."

When Noelle used to have bad days, she took five-mile walks with her dog, or strolled with her husband, something they did regularly when they first started dating.

"I walked through half of Boston with my dog," she said. "We used to walk every single day and go on adventures and I think now, slowly losing the ability to walk has been challenging because I've lost that aspect of my life. That was self-care for me. It gave me space to listen to my own thoughts or listen to music."

These days, she often uses a scooter to replace walking on foot and to use when she goes shopping. Noelle said her husband "said his greatest thing that he loves to see is to see me smile and show people that I'm rocking it. That is our family motto, to rock, no matter what the difficulty that day."

She's also added a device called an L300-go—which provides electrical stimulation to leg muscles to help her walk—to her routine. "That's allowed me to slowly walk further and more safely and has given me more independence."

In spite of rocking her scooter or her L300-go, Noelle said there are days when she laments what she's lost: "I don't have the career I want, but what it has given me is the ability to be more flexible in life, to be more present with my children, to be more present with my husband."

To new MS patients, Noelle says: "Whatever you're feeling or going through, it's okay. Whatever you're experiencing, day-to-day, minute-to-minute, I hear you. I feel you. Those feelings are valid. I think that sometimes, especially on the bad days, your self worth and what's going on, especially when you're going through a flare, sometimes the loneliness kicks in. These feelings will pass."

Resources

National Multiple Sclerosis Society:
https://www.nationalmssociety.org/

Find MS Physicians:
https://www.nationalmssociety.org/resources/get-support/
find-doctors-and-resources/healthcare-provider-guide

Becoming a National MS Society MS Activist:
https://www.nationalmssociety.org/how-you-can-help/
get-involved/advocate/become-an-ms-activist

Multiple Sclerosis Association of America: https://mymsaa.org/

National Institutes of Health, Multiple Sclerosis page:
https://www.nccih.nih.gov/health/multiple-sclerosis

European Committee for Treatment and Research in Multiple
Sclerosis: https://ectrims.eu/

Affordable Care Act for people with multiple sclerosis:
https://www.nationalmssociety.org/resources/financial-
planning/health-insurance/individual-insurance#:~:text=Many%20
people%20living%20with%20multiple,Care%20Act%20pro-
hibits%20such%20restrictions.

Americans with Disabilities Act (ADA): https://www.ada.gov/

International Journal of Environmental Research and Public
Health, "Stigma, Discrimination and Disclosure of the Diagnosis of
Multiple Sclerosis in the Workplace:"
https://pmc.ncbi.nlm.nih.gov/articles/PMC9367867/

U.S. Department of Transportation, traveling with disabilities:
https://www.transportation.gov/individuals/aviation-consumer-
protection/traveling-disability

U.S. Department of Transportation, air travel for those with
disabilities: https://www.transportation.gov/airconsumer

Amtrak (railroad) transportation for those with disabilities:
https://www.amtrak.com/accessible-travel-services

Uncomfortably Numb 2
CONTRIBUTORS

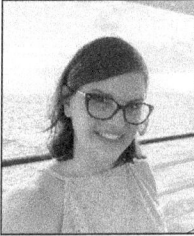

Dianne B., diagnosed with MS in 2013, is a Massachusetts resident, wife, and mom. She loves all things sparkly and indulges her sweet tooth whenever possible. Learn more about the central Massachusetts MS support group she co-leads at instagram.com/-milford_ms_group.

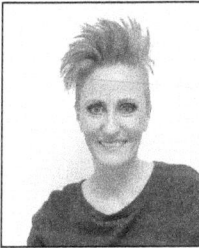

Paige Butas posts videos under the name MS Fighter 101 on TikTok. Learn more at tiktok.com/@msfighter101.

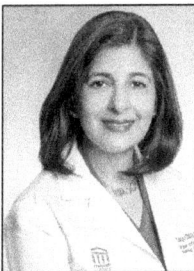

Dr. Tanuja Chitnis is the Cindy Larsen Chugg Distinguished Chair in Neurology at the Brigham and Women's Hospital and is a professor of neurology at Harvard Medical School. She is also the founding director of the Mass General Brigham Pediatric Multiple Sclerosis Center at Massachusetts General Hospital. She has published over 300 peer-reviewed articles in the MS and neuroimmunological diseases field and has received funding awards from the Department of Defense, the National MS Society, and other foundations to support her work. Learn more at brighammscenter.org/about/ms-center-staff/tanuja-chitnis.

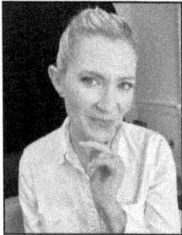

Noelle Connolly is a licensed clinical social worker and a married mother of three who has been living with MS since she was 17. She is determined to change the stigma in society about chronic illness and using mobility aids. Learn more at instagram.com/ms.living-balanced.

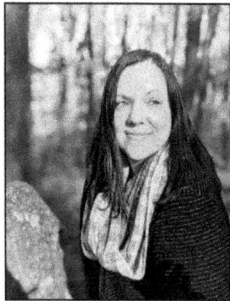

Elissa Grossell Dickey is an author of thrilling, romantic fiction with chronic illness representation, the bestselling *The Speed of Light* (an Amazon First Reads pick) and *Iris in the Dark*. Though she grew up among the lakes and trees of northern Minnesota, Elissa now lives on the South Dakota prairie with her husband and children. A former journalist, she now works as the communications and marketing director for her local public school district. Elissa shared her own personal story living with multiple sclerosis as a past contributor to the National Multiple Sclerosis Society's blog. Learn more at elissadickey.com.

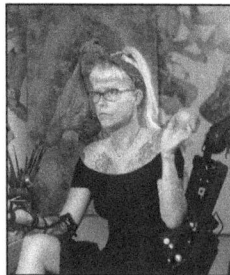

Lydia Emily is an artist and MS advocate living in California with her family. A spokesperson for the National Multiple Sclerosis Society, her artwork—including murals in four American states—raises awareness about MS and other social and political causes. The subject of the documentary *The Art of Rebellion*, Lydia Emily also published a memoir, *The Art of Hope*, about her life with multiple sclerosis. Learn more at lydiaemily.com.

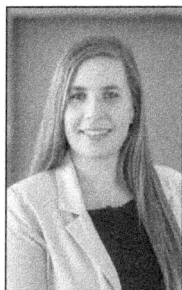

Laura Hoch has been with the National Multiple Sclerosis Society since 2018 and currently serves as associate vice president for state advocacy and policy. She holds a Bachelor of Science in political science and Spanish from the State University of New York at Oneonta and a Master of Public Administration with a concentration in applied politics from The American University.

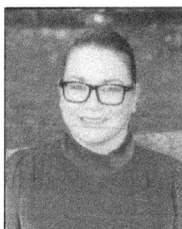

Sarah Quezada is a MSfit, a term she created to embrace her MS while still laughing at herself while living with MS. She lives with her family in California. They love to travel. She routinely eats all the good colors out of candy boxes before lovingly handing them back to her kids to enjoy. Learn more at MSfitmomma.com.

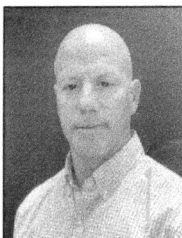

Eddy Tabit is vice president of operations for Simplified Clinical Data Systems. He is also a trustee for the Greater New England Chapter of the National Multiple Sclerosis Society. Eddy lives on the New Hampshire seacoast where he stays active while living with MS.

Acknowledgments

I owe many people thanks for their efforts in making this guide a reality. I want to express my gratitude to:

Nancy Cleary, founder of Wyatt-MacKenzie Publishing, for this gem of an idea to create a book for newly-diagnosed patients. This is something I wish I had when I learned I had MS. I really hope the stories collected in this volume can help people.

Lori Espino, the president of the Greater New England chapter of the National Multiple Sclerosis Society, for connecting me to so many people whose stories add depth and nuance to this guide. Lori has been an invaluable resource for me not just as a writer, but as a friend.

My contributors were wildly generous with their time and their hearts when they not only accepted my invitation to respond to questions but offered incredibly thoughtful and intensely personal stories about their experiences with MS. Thank you to my fellow MS patients Dianne B., Paige Butas, Noelle Connolly, Elissa Grossell Dickey, Lydia Emily, Sarah Quezada, and Eddy Tabit. I am likewise grateful for the time and effort put forth by Dr. Tanuja Chitnis, a specialist in pediatric MS, and Laura Hoch of the National Multiple Sclerosis Society, with whom I've worked to advocate for public policies and laws.

One of my personal heroes in my MS journey also needs a shout out: Dr. Jonathan Zurawski, my stellar neurologist at Mass General Brigham, who actively listens to my concerns, provides excellent care, and is an indefatigable cheerleader for me and for all of us living with MS. It's my wish that everyone has a neurologist like him.

I would like to thank the many selfless MS social media influencers and writers who chronicle their experiences which enable the rest of us to feel seen and understood. You help to create a community where everyone's voice is important.

Thank you to the members of Taco Salad, the Bike MS team formed in 2023, which raised thousands of dollars for the National Multiple Sclerosis Society for the Great Maine Getaway event. This team includes close family friends, my husband, and my two sons. Many thanks, my dudes.

Finally, I'd like to thank my family for their patience, for their love, and for being ferociously protective even when I resist your help. Specifically, I'm grateful for my husband Scott, who seeks to help me in any way he can and who accompanies me to many National Multiple Sclerosis Society and book-related events. You're my rock.

◆